-12

HOW GOLF
CAN SAVE YOUR LIFE

HOW GOLF CAN SAVE YOUR LIFE

DREW MILLARD

ABRAMS PRESS, NEW YORK

Library of Congress Control Number: 2022948255

ISBN: 978-1-4197-5757-0
eISBN: 978-1-64700-444-6

Printed and bound in the United States
10 9 8 7 6 5 4 3 2 1

ABRAMS The Art of Books
195 Broadway, New York, NY 10007
abramsbooks.com

CONTENTS

INTRODUCTION

If there's one thing golf demands above all else, it's honesty.

—Jack Nicklaus, *Golf My Way*

IN THE SPRING of 2020, I was laid off from my job. I edited feature articles for a website, and the website no longer had any use for my services because the website itself had ceased to exist. This happened, more or less, as a result of COVID-19 and the economic downturn that policymakers predicted would accompany it. The entire thing sucked.

This was right around the time that lockdowns throughout the nation caused the vast majority of nonessential businesses to close their doors, meaning that I suddenly had a surfeit of free time but not much to actually do with it.

There was, however, golf. I have a deep emotional connection to this silly sport. It has been there for me when I was at the lowest point in my life, and it has stayed with me as I've grown into the person I am now. I spent the majority of the early pandemic's head-spinning days going to Hillandale Golf Course in Durham, North Carolina, where I was living at the time. Golf was one of the few things outside my own home that offered safety and a feeling of spiritual wholeness. I played it almost constantly, and I quickly noticed that I wasn't the only one who'd decided to hit the links in the face of COVID. Though the course had always been a beloved local golf institution, it was more crowded and vibrant than I'd ever seen.

Where I'd once been able to park my car, check in at the pro shop, and immediately tee off, I now had to wait for a free tee time to open up, puttering around the practice green scanning for my fellow regulars amid a sea of new faces.

At every course I went to during that time, I'd meet people who'd just found their way into golf—millennials, mostly, underemployed and a little bored, who began aimlessly ambling around the course just to kill time, only to discover the game's addictive properties. Many of them were not, strictly speaking, very good. But the thing about golf is that often your lack of mastery only compels you. When there aren't any expectations, every move you make feels like a bold step forward. That's an incredibly freeing notion.

I have a theory that for millions of people, coronavirus forced upon us an unexpected reckoning, or perhaps a reevaluation, when it came to how we spent our time. Within this newly meditative period, we realized that the idea of "being busy" had become an end unto itself, part of this fake narrative that everyone was equal and that if you simply hustled hard enough, you would distinguish yourself and be rewarded.

And yet when the hustle faucet got turned off, society seemed to reward its victors and punish its losers even more arbitrarily than it had before. Some people—especially those in tech, real estate, or the newly minted industry of speculating on GameStop stock or NFTs—made out great, while others were sent toward or even past the brink of disaster, experiencing food and housing insecurity, a lack of medical care, or jobs that forced them into harm's way in order to keep getting a paycheck. Stimulus checks or not, the whole thing was enough to make you want to retreat from the world.

Again: During the first months of the pandemic, millions of people came to golf for millions of reasons. According to the National Golf Foundation, 6.2 million people either took up the game or returned to it in 2020, which included an 8 percent increase in new female golfers. Those people stuck around, or at least so it seems: By the end of July 2021, Americans had played 16.1 percent more rounds of golf than they had by the end of the previous July. Given that this was at a time when many of us had been vaccinated and America was much more open than it had been the year before, this suggests to me that golf's newfound popularity was a product of coronavirus, not an isolated symptom. The pandemic had sparked the golf bug in people, but once their eyes were opened to its numerous joys, they kept playing even as the normalcy of the world around them ebbed and flowed like the tides off Kiawah Island.

This wasn't the first time we've turned to golf amid a crisis. During the twin calamities that were World War I and the Spanish flu pandemic, President Woodrow Wilson urged soldiers awaiting deployment to play golf in order to get exercise without becoming sick; one newspaper reported that members of golf clubs in and around Portland, Oregon, had "declare[d] their immunity from" Spanish flu due to the fact that "golf tends toward health." OK, so they weren't exactly following the science, to borrow a coronavirus-era phrase, but you've got to appreciate their enthusiasm. During the Great Depression, a surplus of then-unused urban space led to a semi-out-of-nowhere interest in miniature golf, whose courses could be built anywhere and out of anything, as long as you laid some artificial turf over it all. American soldiers stuck in German POW camps during World War II played the game on makeshift holes using clubs donated by the Red Cross. For all the hay that's made about golf being elitist and inaccessible, it's remarkable the degree to which people can and have figured out ways to play it pretty much anywhere.

It's golf's ability to foster ingenuity under duress, I think, that animated what I'm going to call the Great Coronavirus Golf Revival. For some context, the last time the sport saw an explosion in popularity, it was largely due to the emergence of Tiger Woods. While there had been countless professional golfers who were cool—Lee Trevino got his start as a country club cart attendant who hustled members on the side; John Daly became a folk hero for being a hard-drinking, long-hitting dude with a mullet; and the wisecracking Chi Chi Rodríguez was so cool that Devo put him on the cover of its first album—but Tiger was the first golfer to bring an imprimatur of cool to golf itself. For over a decade, he was the sport's center of gravity, and despite late-career scandals, back injuries that eventually limited his ability to compete, and a car crash that nearly ended his life, as I write this in 2022, there's still no one who's managed to eclipse his fame. He's not the dominant force he once was, and the fact that the sport's most well-known player doesn't actually compete that much has left professional golf in a really weird place. Right now, most famous pros can be categorized as (A) oddball underdogs whose charisma can garner them little factional fandoms who freak out whenever they win some random tournament every sixteen months, or (B) flawless players who made some sort of Faustian bargain in which they traded their personalities for absolute golf perfection. There are enough players in category A to keep golf interesting to watch, but without a single figure as its face, it lacks the ability it once had to bring people to the game.

It was this absence of a Tiger-like force, though, that helped make room for golfers at the game's deeply amateur, hobbyist margins to reshape it in their own image from the ground up. Golf fashion, once relegated to the realm of mall department stores, went nuts, with niche golf clothing popping up all over to inject both style and levity into a look that was once defined by ill-fitting khakis and bland, draping polo shirts. One company, Malbon, worked with Nike to adapt iconic Air Jordan silhouettes into golf shoes; another, Metalwood Studio, mined the aesthetics of golf's past to create clothes that managed to be both genuinely fashion-forward and somehow an implicit parody of the big-box fare of yore.

This penchant for remixing and reimagining found its way into golf bags as well. The pandemic saw the ascent of the minimalist golf movement, whose practitioners favor short sets, usually consisting of one or two woods, maybe a hybrid, three or four irons, a wedge or two, and a putter—well below the conventional fourteen that most people bag these days—and carried their sticks rather than drove a cart. On Instagram, these players post photos of their setups, trading compliments about having bags that feature classic (and now inexpensive) clubs from the mid-2000s, whose time-tested durability and quality are as valuable on the course as any thousand-dollar set of irons. As a whole, the idea of minimalist golf represents golf as an exercise in simplicity: walking the course, enjoying nature with no distractions—including unnecessary clubs—and being thrifty while you do it.

I want to make it clear, though, that this is not a "pandemic book." It's just that I happened to write a good chunk of these essays while the world was in the thick of COVID, and so things bled through. Looking back, it's remarkable how much my life was dominated by the rituals of mask-wearing, hand-sanitizing, basing my social life around when the weather was nice, always checking infection statistics online, and becoming maddeningly familiar with various videoconferencing software systems. It provided for an undercurrent of deep melancholy that you may encounter in some chapters, because the world had suddenly changed, and I and everyone I love were being forced to change with it. Still, while coronavirus may have provided the context for much of this book's events, its content was inspired by golf and golf alone.

By the way: On the off chance that you're reading this in, say, the year 2123, the coronavirus was so pervasive and made so many people sick (or worse) that for a while in the early 2020s, it was the primary filter through which people viewed their entire existence. It was sort of exciting to go through in the way any tragedy can be, because it felt like we were all living in historic times, but it also turned out that, due to this historic event making it so that people had to spend lots of time inside, it was fairly boring on a day-to-day level. The times that coronavirus was not boring was when you had it, in which case it was either annoying or scary, depending on the severity of your case, or when it caused someone you knew to die, in which case it was just devastating. Even so, there was a lot of boredom, and the nature of that boredom encouraged lots and lots of people to pick up a golf club or fourteen.

My hope is that reading this will do two things for you. First, I hope my own story can serve as a guide that helps you understand what golf means to you—to reconsider your own experiences with the game and place them in conversation with the rest of your life so that both come out more rewarding. And second, if you don't play golf, I want you to give golf a shot. It's not like golf is this magic thing that will unlock every secret of existence or anything, but it's both mentally and physically stimulating, a deep game with so much to offer that it's almost impossible *not* to play it on your own terms.

That said, I'm not picky about whether or not you play. If you do, I hope you approach it with an open mind and an appreciation of its idiosyncrasies. If you don't, I've tried to keep the specialized terminology to a minimum, and there's a glossary in the back that covers the basics if you ever feel lost. Because really, I wrote this book for you. Don't tell the golfers that, because I wrote it for them, too. But despite what anyone may say, golf is for everyone. I want to be your tour guide as you enter this world. I'll tell you about the game's history, rules, and customs in the hope of demystifying them, using my own experiences as a jumping-off point. Golf has also changed the way I think about the world, and my personal philosophies have also impacted the way I think about golf. As Jack Nicklaus says above, golf demands honesty, so I've tried to be honest about myself here. Most of the conversations recounted in this book were unrecorded; some are based on detailed notes I took in the minutes after having them, while other quotes appear with the blessing of those to whom they are attributed. As for the stuff drawing from the distant past, well, I did my best.

With all of that in mind, I'd like to tell you about the worst thing that ever happened to me.

Chapter One

HOW GOLF SAVED MY LIFE

IT DIDN'T START when I rear-ended that guy's used Mercedes, but that was probably the straw that broke the camel's back. The camel, unfortunately, was already holding way too many expensive clothes I'd bought with my credit card, because that's what I thought people in Los Angeles were supposed to do. It was the spring of 2016, and I was feeling alone and like I was buckling under the weight of every decision I'd ever made. Had I even consciously chosen to ask my boss to relocate me here from New York? Whose idea was it for me to quit my editing job not even a year after I got here, to write freelance articles for the same company that used to pay my health insurance? Did I, of my own volition, take the assignment to cover that Young Thug concert last night, and what did any of this have to do with sleeping only three hours before having to wake up to write a feature about trends in vaporizer technology for a trade magazine? Things were just happening to me, like I'd abdicated custody over my own life after that panic attack two years ago sent me running from my desk straight to the doctor's office, where I announced, loudly and without any hint of self-consciousness, that I was dying.

But now, whoever I'd left in charge was having a heated argument on the side of Melrose Avenue with some guy who was demanding that I cough up $750 to fix a bumper that had already been scratched to hell before I knocked him at maybe ten miles an hour. The guy leveled with me: Unless I paid him right now, he was going to get the insurance companies involved so he could get a new body piece or two and send my premiums shooting up in the process.

The next day, I sent the guy his money and admitted defeat. I called my parents and asked them if I could come back home. I was broke and miserable; I needed to get out of this place, this life. They bought me a plane ticket and told me everything would be OK. I didn't believe them, but they were right. My dad had just decided to run for Congress, and even though he wasn't going to win, I could tell everyone in LA that I was leaving to help with his campaign, until I was ready to come clean about what was actually going on.

Once I made it back to my folks' place in western North Carolina, I barricaded myself in my childhood bedroom, the little black dog I'd adopted in LA tucked into my chest. Nora was the best thing that came out of my time on the West Coast. The rescue group had found her living under a house, taking care of a litter of puppies, so she was used to guarding the defenseless. Seeing as my parents live in the middle of nowhere, the only things around that counted as threats in her eyes were the squirrels she could make out through a bend in the metal shutters of my room, and my mom when she'd open the door unannounced to see how I was doing, maybe gently suggest that I go see a doctor or something. I appreciated the sentiment—on both my mom's part and the dog's—but doing things, even thinking thoughts, was too much to handle.

Instead, I lay in bed, shifting my focus from the gray walls to the navy carpet and back. With the lights off and the shades drawn, the gradation wasn't much, but it complemented my range of emotions.

Half a decade later, I can now confidently say this: Working in online media seriously fucked with my head. It's an industry that rewards people who get the most pairs of eyeballs on the stories they write, regardless of their quality. And then the brain rewards these people by firing off a dopamine rush in response to the instant feedback that comes after pressing "publish," and watching the traffic pile up and getting responses from readers in real time on social media.

The high from this dopamine rush feels so good that you do not care whether people are reading your stuff because they love it or because you've pissed them off. And this can end up rewiring your brain to believe that it is extremely good that thousands of people you've never met are mad at you. I know this one guy in Toronto who googled himself every day, and kept doing wilder and wilder stuff to keep people talking. Ended up getting a whole true-crime podcast made about him. Also ten years for cocaine trafficking. "Don't worry," he told me right before his sentencing, "it's *Canadian* prison." Now he spends all day sewing face masks for $60 a week, then fishing, then lifting weights, then typing out letters on a computer that isn't hooked up to the internet. It took a little trial and error, but the dude's got it all figured out.

For me, the internet created a remove between my private self, who tried to do the right thing, and my professional self, who existed in an environment where conventional morality was just another thing holding the web traffic numbers down, along with constantly shifting social media algorithms, and Stewart from sales saying we shouldn't write a takedown about Skip Bayless, because he was *this close* to working out a branded content deal with ESPN, so please delete that post immediately. On top of the crush of that dissonance was the weight of all the mental energy I expended just trying to get by. The writing gigs I was taking back then were in low supply but high demand, meaning that as a freelance writer, I found myself filing multiple articles per week, sometimes multiple articles per day, at the highest level I could muster, in order to maintain some semblance of an income.

When I wasn't actively writing, I was coming up with ideas for articles whose worth would be measured by how many people read them. For every pitch that got picked up, there were probably five that got rejected, meaning I had a 20 percent success rate of guessing what was inside the head of an editor who was trying to guess what was inside the heads of millions of anonymous internet people. Mostly, my process involved looking at a thing that had already happened, trying to predict the consensus opinion about that thing, and then racing against probably twenty other writers to articulate that opinion first. I did not find it particularly significant that Kanye West rapped about being on antidepressants, or that Teva sandals were back in style, or that Justin Bieber was not a particularly conscientious monkey owner—all of which were brief pop culture concerns during the mid-2010s that I issued opinions on. But I told myself I cared about all of them, and maybe I even believed it.

At some point there in my childhood bedroom, my sense of melancholy broke, like a fever does, and I began to see things as they were. It's like I'd stepped out for some air, lost track of time, and come back home a couple of years later to find cigarette butts and sawdust on the floor and a family of squirrels trying to make an omelet on the stove, unaware that they'd somehow managed to make the toilet catch fire. The shock tends to spur you to act. So I peeled back the covers of my bed, oozed onto the floor and into my car, and drove myself to an urgent care clinic. It didn't take a rocket scientist to figure out I was experiencing a severe depressive episode, but it did take a doctor to get me on some medication that might help remedy the situation. Antidepressants alone, he told me, weren't going to cut it with a case like mine, and I agreed—my goal wasn't to make the rut I was in little less uncomfortable; the idea was to transcend the rut altogether. I asked him if he could recommend a therapist; he referred me to someone who ran a practice out of the sitting room of her cabin. Then he told me the thing that changed my life forever: I needed to start getting some exercise.

Now, as a rule, I do not exercise. The only way I can get myself moving my body vigorously for a prolonged period is if that vigorous movement is coincidental to some other thing that I'm already doing. Like playing basketball, or running from a bear. But as much as I hated exercise, I hated the way that I felt even more. Too often, we become what we do for work, but my work had put me in front of this doctor. I'd spent so many years trying to professionally please others that I barely knew who I was anymore. But I was once a person who did things for myself—I must have been—and then I remembered.

"I used to play golf," I told the doctor. "I guess I could get back into it, if that counts." I'd played a little as a kid, and had been on my high school golf team, but I was never very good at it. I was one of those teenagers who'd go to sleep at night and wake up an inch taller, and my brain was always trying to recalibrate my motor functions for that day's body. I was clumsy, prone to fits of nerves, and self-conscious in all the ways teenagers are. This did not add up to a particularly illustrious junior golf career, but hey, at least it meant I had an old set of clubs laying around.

I wasn't sure where they were, exactly; I hadn't seen them in a long time. I'd gone off to college, where I'd gotten into DJing at the radio station and reading Marxist theory, as one does. I joined a punk band, also as one does, then quit the punk band when I graduated and moved to New York. I got a job at a place called VICE Media, writing about hip-hop. I entered a milieu of bookish hipsters, the kind of crowd where mentioning that you'd played golf in high school was a way of demonstrating how uncool you used to be and, by extension, how cool you had become. As I got more and more into my new life, there came a point where I stopped thinking about the sport altogether, and by my mid-twenties, the fact that I'd once golfed at all felt like a half-forgotten dream. But now life had worn me down to the nub, and I desperately needed something that could build me back up again. I needed exercise. The doctor said that golf was exercise.

That afternoon, I was in my parents' basement, searching for my old clubs in the unfinished storage area under the stairs, navigating an obstacle course of wire shelves overflowing with dusty boxes full of Christmas decorations and relics from my childhood, each with a label denoting the contents and era neatly printed in Magic Marker by my mother. The clubs were already a decade old when my dad bought them for me back when I was fourteen and settling into an adult-ish body. The irons were flecked with rust; the fairway woods sported a flat sole and ultra-low profile that years of R&D had innovated into obsolescence many times over. The newest thing in the bag was my putter, a rusted piece of metal that my uncle, a lifelong tinkerer who operated a side business making custom pool cues, had designed in his den and built in his garage with the same milling machine he used for his cues. In the place of a traditional putter shaft, he'd jammed the lower half of a pool cue into his creation and called it a day. It was all jumbled and mismatched, but it was what the doctor ordered.

Next came the golf course, the same one I'd played a million and a half times back in high school, tucked into the side of a hill thirteen minutes away from my folks', eleven if you gun it on the straightaway past my old middle school and get lucky with the light at the intersection. I let my golf bag rest by the practice green and walked up the stone steps leading to the clubhouse, an old log cabin with thin carpet on the floors and a busted cigarette machine from the Eisenhower administration sitting next to the counter. The course itself was built in 1916, and the golf pro, a silver-haired Southerner with the sort of paunch that conveniently helps older golfers place their hands the ideal distance from their center of gravity as they swing, told me that the place was celebrating its hundredth anniversary by waiving its $500 initiation fee for new members, so I could either give him $12 to go out and play nine or pay $50 for a membership and play all the golf I wanted for a month. I went with that one and gave him an extra 10 bucks for a dozen used golf balls from a bucket that had charmingly been labeled RENTAL BALLS—after all, once I inevitably hit one into a pond, the course could just fish it out and sell it again.

The course was exactly as I remembered it. Five of its holes spoked out from the practice green, while the other four wrapped around them to form a squishy wheel. Hole one was a short par 5, its fairway lined with trees to the left and split horizontally by a creek off in the distance. I teed up my ball and took a couple of tentative practice swings. A golf swing is a rapid, fluid motion with a lot of moving parts. It's a hard thing to visualize while simultaneously executing, which is a roundabout way of saying that when I actually tried to hit my ball off the tee, I nearly missed it.

Hitting a golf ball for the first time in a long time isn't so much like riding a bicycle again as it is like riding a unicycle for the first time. You know how to pedal, yes, that's familiar, but you're missing a bunch of stuff that should feel normal, like handlebars and that other wheel. Then you realize: You've got to provide the stuff that's missing, a sense of rhythm and balance that can only be learned with time. There are a million little questions to ask yourself at every stage of the swing, and the answers have a monumental impact on where the ball goes. The trick is to know the answers so well that they're etched into your muscle memory and the entire process is subconscious. Two shots in, I was only halfway to the creek I should have already cleared. I decided to stop trying to remember all the mechanical nonsense and just swing, hoping that if I killed the noise, some signal might shine through.

You recognize a good shot from the second you make contact. When you hit a ball in the sweet spot of the club, it creates vibrations that to your ears register as a firm *thwack*, but to your body register like an endorphin rush in reverse, this sense of joyous peace that shoots up the club and into your hands, through your arms to your chest, and up into your brain. I took a breath, squinted, and let my body take over. Then I heard the *thwack*, I felt the rush, and I knew my third shot was perfect even before my eye caught it in the distance, flying over the creek.

As I watched the ball roll to a stop in the middle of the fairway, I experienced my first flash of true happiness in months. Suddenly, the world was bright, alive, full of possibility. I remembered that the word "verdant" existed, and that someone must have invented it to describe the fairway on which I was now strolling. The pungency of a nearby Bradford pear tree hit my nose. I made eye contact with a squirrel stuffing its mouth with berries and briefly contemplated its interior world.

The ball was resting on a plateau maybe a football field's length away from the green. A par was within reach. All I had to do now was hit the green and make the putt. I was so excited that I cranked my pitching wedge way too far back, nearly banging myself on the shoulder, and brought it back down so hard I ended up digging an otter's tail into the earth. Absolutely terrible shot, but every millisecond I got to watch it hang in the air, only to land short of the green, felt like a gift.

I'd fallen in love with golf all over again. I'm talking climbing a mountain, jumping over the moon, standing outside golf's window holding a boom box levels of love. I loved it so much that I even loved how much I sucked at it.

You create feedback loops when you play—you do a thing, see the effect, and if the effect is bad, adjust accordingly, then do some more adjustments based on whatever new bad thing crops up. After I figured out how to make consistent contact with the ball, every shot began screaming toward my target, only to have a change of heart mid-flight and jerk violently to the left. I moved my feet farther apart in the hope that it would do something. It did, but the thing was bad: Now the ball was taking sharp right turns. Over the coming weeks, I shifted my stance so frequently that I think I accidentally learned how to do the jitterbug. But for the first time since I'd lost all my serotonin somewhere in Los Angeles, I was doing something.

When you're seventeen, not knowing who you are will drive you nuts. It's why teens love slamming doors in their parents' faces and then shaving their eyebrows while waiting for the Manic Panic they just put in their hair to dry. But at twenty-seven, it's freeing. You realize there's always time to shake off your old identity, cast yourself in a new light, make a hard break from what isn't working, and meander off in whichever direction feels right. I'd once been a writer who lived in Los Angeles and stayed up late going to rap concerts. Now I was just some dude in the middle of nowhere who was figuring it all out by going to therapy and playing a lot of golf.

Clearly, golf is not the only reason I recovered from my breakdown. But on both a physical and mental level, golf primed the pump. I was once again an agent in the cycle of cause and effect, one in which the results mattered less than the realization that the will my depression had robbed me of was slowly returning. It gave me a reason for being, beyond the professional, beyond even the personal. Sucking at golf was a calling.

• • •

Soon enough, I started doing more things. Like canvassing suburbia with my dad, trying to convince neighborhoods full of Republicans to vote for him, the sacrificial Democrat of that election cycle. I watched as he debated his opponent at a craft brewery, catered by Chick-fil-A, and felt my soul deflate afterward in the bathroom as I heard one guy at the sink say to another, "Great debate. Too bad that Democrat ain't got a chance in hell."

Even though this was only a few years ago, it truly was a different historical epoch. There was an optimism that things could still happen in an orderly and incremental way, that Hillary Clinton was going to become the president and our reward for voting her in was that we could check out of politics until the midterms and that, somehow, things would all be a little better than they were when we'd last checked in. But life doesn't work like that. Sitting back and watching the world happen is how you end up depressed and living with your parents. You've got to put in the work, and it's the work itself that has meaning. Golf taught me that, but only after my dad lost in the landslide that also got Donald Trump elected did I understand that this lesson is universal.

I made it my mission to gather every object I might need to golf. Every thrift store in America has a big bucket hiding near the back wall stuffed with oodles of used golf clubs, indiscriminately priced at a quarter each, and the trick is to go to the same one every day until something worth buying shows up. That's how I got my second set of golf clubs for 20 bucks—$2.50 for the irons and woods, $17.50 for a bag that still had a few balls inside.

Half a decade of black T-shirts, overpriced skinny jeans, and frequent relocations had left me with no golf attire to speak of. At first, I stole polo shirts from my dad, who's one of those guys who finds one type of shirt that looks good on him and buys it in every color. But the problem is he likes those shirts, and also I wanted to move out at some point. Back to the thrift store I went. Former PGA star Greg Norman, a bronzed Australian nicknamed "the Great White Shark," who looks like a cross between Woody Harrelson and Gary Busey and used to win tournaments while wearing a cowboy hat, may be famous for being the top player in the world before Tiger Woods came around. But to me, he's the guy who lent his name to a clothing company, Greg Norman Collection, whose every product has the texture of a chenille blanket and looks like the year 1995. I have no idea why the golf dads of Polk County, North Carolina, decided en masse to get rid of all their old Greg Norman shirts in the summer of 2016, but now I own them.

That fall, I started writing again, and I enjoyed it. I poured my soul into a profile of an aging porn mogul and got so into it I even interviewed the guy's antiques dealer. I started covering

North Carolina politics, which meant both reporting on goings-on in the state legislature and hanging out in the middle of nowhere with a couple of hundred anarchists who were carrying sticks and looking for a KKK rally to bust up. I started collecting old records and wrote about that, too. The pay wasn't great, but it was enough to finally move me out of my parents' house and into a garage apartment four hours away in Durham.

The Raleigh-Durham area is absolutely lousy with courses, and I made it my personal mission to play all of them. I started out exploring the local goat tracks—under-maintained munis with cheapo prices and misguided layouts that try to squeeze eighteen holes into a space fit for fifteen—then worked my way up to venues meant for golf's middle class, courses attached to bland housing developments that can actually afford to hire a maintenance crew. When I could pay for it, I'd splurge on a late-afternoon round at a true diamond, like N.C. State's bajillion-dollar facility designed by Arnold Palmer (of golf and iced-tea-plus-lemonade renown), which pulls triple duty as a wildlife preserve and a laboratory for the school's turf management program. You play the goat tracks to lodge scores that boost your self-esteem, the mid-tier ones to get an accurate gauge of your ability, and the diamonds to see what you're made of. Try hitting a gap wedge into the wind on a downhill par 3 with a triangle-shaped green guarded by a fox who's ready to attack if your ball lands near her patch of overgrown brush, and you'll know what I mean.

Golf courses themselves are living beings. During morning rounds, the dew on the grass makes everything almost look blue, and on every green, I can see fleeting, anonymous histories of putts in the form of little dry lines running toward the hole. In the early evenings, that moisture migrates into the air. I become a little delirious, flirt with heatstroke, convinced I'm chasing the sun with every shot I hit. In the spring, a course's greens seem to inhale the fresh air, and by mid-June, they've become stuffed, soft, and spongy, and ready to catch any shot that comes their way. During the winters, they harden, as if scabbing over so that they can heal after months of wear and tear. On especially cold days, they're so unwelcoming that shots bounce off them like they're slabs of concrete.

I got into a rhythm of playing three times a week, four when I had a deadline I wanted to miss. I learned that the equation for making your car smell like something died in it was sweaty golf socks plus heat plus time. I got a new job writing and editing for a new website where we all worked from home and I was able to slink off in the afternoons to squeeze in a quick nine. I began dating someone who lived in New York, and after two years of us flying back and forth to see each other, we got a place together in Durham. I bought a car that I liked enough to not leave socks in it. We got another dog to keep our beloved Nora company, and he—he being Percy, the new dog—started making the new car smell weird, which is more respectable somehow. More good things happened than bad things, or at least I had grown enough to know that the bad things weren't the end of everything. Time passed, and I spent more of it playing golf than most people do.

Most of the time, my local public course was like a town in the Old West, its sparse population made up of a few characters, a couple of drunks, and a sheriff who kept order and occasionally gave golf lessons to children. Then, in the spring of 2020, I took a personal day from work because writing so many articles about coronavirus had given me a panic attack, went to the golf course around lunchtime to help clear my head, and discovered that the ghost town had become a beehive.

It turns out that a nationwide pandemic spread by people inhaling each other's air was bad for a lot of things, but it was great for golf. Golf courses are a bit like restaurants: Sometimes, you can just show up and eat; other times, you need to call ahead. Coronavirus turned every course into a reservation-only affair. Where did these people come from, I wondered, as I watched an old man give putting tips to a couple of frat dudes at the practice green while dodging errant chip shots from the perimeter. On the driving range, a woman pulled the shade down on her baby carriage and began beating balls next to me. We made eye contact, and she shrugged. *Shit happens*, she seemed to say, *and right now, golf is the only shit that's happening*.

She was right. Four weeks later, I got laid off from my job, and so did everyone I worked with. They told us all at once on a conference call, which was cathartic in a trauma-bonding kind of way. If we had all lived in the same city and the world had been normal, we would have gone to a bar and had an Irish wake for our now-defunct publication. Instead, we started a group text where we shared tips about signing up for unemployment, and I booked a tee time for that afternoon. When I got to the course, I left my phone in my car. It was one of those distinctly North Carolina days when the weather's ominously perfect. On the third hole, the wind blew my six-iron shot back on course so that my ball landed ten feet from the pin, leaving me with a putt just easy enough to feel bad about missing. My vision was blurry and I was still rattled from the morning, so missing it is exactly what I did. I finished out the hole, pocketed my ball, shouldered my golf bag, and walked to the next tee.

Chapter Two

HOW GOLF TAUGHT ME ABOUT CREATIVITY

IMAGINE YOU'RE A Scottish farmer. Why are you a farmer, exactly? Well, the year's 1459, so you don't have a lot of options. The printing press in Europe was just invented a couple of decades ago, which means you probably still can't read, and, as a non-noble, your options were to either go off to the big city of St. Andrews and try to make it as a craftsman—good luck with that, buddy—or to stick to the land you grew up on, twenty miles away from the city, working the same plot that your family has tilled for generations, trading a portion of your crops to some rich guy you've never met in exchange for your house and plot. The good news, though, is you live in the relatively comfortable Lowlands, as opposed to up in the mountainous Highlands, where everybody's backward as hell and no one even has pants yet. I mean, it's not like you own any pants, either, but if you saved up enough, you *could* own some pants.

It's a Sunday, and you're supposed to be in church. But it's nice out, and you figure nobody'll notice if you skip out just this once, so you and your neighbor Dawy go to meet your friend Johnne at the center of the village square to head out for a game of golf. Johnne's kind of a weird guy, as far as things go these days. He's a humanist, which means he's already broken from the Catholic Church toward a less oppressive version of Christianity—he's also technically a heretic, but the last time they burned one of those guys was when you were a kid, so while you're worried about the fate of his soul, you're less concerned about his physical safety. Unlike you, Johnne is trying to make a go of it as an artisan, and is the second-most-successful shoewright in town. He's a good guy, always fun to be around, has interesting ideas, and oh man, what the hell, he's got a pair of pants! The hairs on your legs, already bitten by the wind, stand on end in quiet jealousy.

The three of you embark on the short walk toward the coast of the North Sea, where the linksland beckons. Nobody you know actually owns the land they work or the houses they live in, but the links are different. If you knew anything about the outside world, you'd have understood that these green, hilly land formations that exist in a liminal space between the Lowlands and the dunes leading to the beach were a geographic anomaly, distinct to this part of Scotland. But all you know is that they're too windy and bumpy to farm on, so a long time ago, some king declared that the links were for all to use. People go to the links to hunt wild rabbits; Dawy keeps a small flock of sheep and grazes them there as well. He knows all the good spots, where his animals and others have trampled and nibbled upon the grasses until they're short enough to golf on without losing your ball.

Dawy leads you into a nice grassy valley near the sea, where you set your homemade clubs down and get to constructing your course. You've each brought some old fenceposts that you'll place as targets on the greens, working them around in a circle so that you create a hole where your balls will come to rest. The three of you head off in different directions, hoping to lay out one hole each, scouting the links for the widest areas to use as fairway, after which you'll look for rabbit patches, where the short, finely grazed grasses are perfect for putting upon.

Thanks to a tip from Dawy to check past that ridge near the sea, you hit pay dirt: an oblong clearing that's been freshly gnawed up by someone's flock, with two potential greens to the north and one toward the south, nestled right up to a plateau that drops into sandy, scraggly overgrowth. You'll be able to play this hole both forward and backward plus on an angle toward the next tee. For an added challenge, the winds are blowing so hard that you'll have to aim your shots toward the sea if you hope to land them in the fairway, but if the wind's calm or your aim is off, your ball's liable to fly straight into one of the bunkers pockmarking the seaward side of the field, where years of sand have built up to create a treacherous lie from which few could hope to recover gracefully.

You reconvene with your friends to tell them the good news. Dawy was able to lay out a couple of nice holes himself, while Johnne was too busy experimenting with the niblick (a short-range club) you just finished carving for yourself that he never got around to doing his share of the searching. Trousers change a man, you think to yourself, wondering how a pair of trousers might change you.

To be fair, Johnne was taken with the niblick because you did a really good job with it. It's meant for hitting short shots onto the green, or for use in those unfortunate situations where you need to get over and out of a pit of sand, and judging by the shots you hit with it behind your cottage, it's just the tool for the job. Your old niblick tended to get caught in tall grass, which is how it ended up breaking off your shaft and flying into a sand dune a couple of months back. It's probably a wild dog's chew toy at this point. This time around, you're confident that it'll stay put. You're happy to try it out with your two new golf balls, courtesy of Colban, your other neighbor. Colban used to come along with you guys to play, but he gave up the game once King James's edict came down banning golf and telling people to take up archery (if you're gonna have a hobby, it might as well be one that doubles as training in case of an invasion, the king figured). Even though most people ignored it—it's not like the king's gonna personally schlep all over Scotland and enforce his dumb new order—Colban's a rule follower from way back, so he dutifully gave up the game. Still, it was awfully nice of him to give you the balls, especially seeing as he made them from the knucklebones of his sheep that died unexpectedly and you didn't even give him a bereavement gift.

Before you embark upon your five holes, you compose some rules. There are some horses grazing around you, and in order to discourage Dawy (the group prankster) from trying to bounce a ball off their hooves, Johnne suggests you enact a one-stroke penalty for striking an animal. Remembering the shining that Johnne took to your niblick, you declare a moratorium on borrowing clubs.

Normally, lending a club to a friend wouldn't be a big deal, because it's not like any of you have any nice stuff.

The Black Death did a real number on the whole "inexorable march of progress" thing, so you and everyone else you know end up carving things like golf clubs and balls by hand, using the tools you have at your disposal. Nobody, including you, has any idea what a golf club's actually supposed to look like, because standardized golf equipment is still a few hundred years away. Instead, you all tinker in your spare time, basing your own clubs on things already in the world. And I'm gonna be honest: Your longnose, your spoon, and your cleek (the equivalents of a modern driver, fairway wood, and putter, respectively) all suck. They look like actual clubs, like the kind a caveman would use, but with some flattish parts for hitting the ball straight. Dawy, meanwhile, based his clubs off his shepherd's crook, and crazy-ass Johnne made some wooden shoes that he jammed onto the hilt of some old spears he had lying around.

But while carving your new niblick, you hit upon a revelation: If the point of this club is to cut through the grass, why not model it after your scythe? You took care to give it as sharp a bottom edge as possible, angling its face upward so that when you sweep the ground, you launch the ball in the air, turf be damned. You have no way of knowing this, but you've just invented a really primitive version of the modern golf club. What you most definitely know, however, is that fancy-pants Johnne does *not* get to use your goddamn niblick, and you tell him as such. He then wagers his trousers against your niblick that he'll have a lower score on more holes than you. You accept, and even though your niblick gets you out of trouble over and over again, neither of you considered that ten is an even number of holes and you end the round with a tie. You offer to carve a replica of your niblick for Johnne if he stitches a pair of trousers together for you out of old shoe leather. He accepts, you go home as friends, and you've accidentally become the first professional golf club manufacturer. Three years later, you die defending your village against foreign raiders because you were so busy playing golf that you never learned how to shoot a bow and arrow. The end.

• • •

As far as anyone can tell, this is how early golf looked. People didn't build golf courses as much as they found them on the Scottish links, they crafted crazy-looking golf clubs out of blocks of wood, and they made up the actual rules of the game right before they started playing. We also know that the game was popular back then thanks in part to a 1457 law passed by the Parliament of Scotland's King James II banning golf along with soccer. (As you might have guessed by the way I wrote about it, modern historians think that few people actually followed that particular edict.)

Unlike, say, basketball or baseball, golf doesn't have an origin story. There's no one guy who woke up one day and said, "I am inventing a new game, and it will be called golf." Instead, the sport evolved over time, with one generation building upon what previous ones had left them, adapting it for their own particular time and circumstances. But generally, we give golf a creation myth, claiming that it was started by Scottish farmers in the late Middle Ages in the area around St. Andrews, which was then a popular destination for religious pilgrimages. In the 1500s, it became the site of the first permanent golf course, which someone eventually thought to call the Old Course at St. Andrews. Much like Stonehenge or weighted blankets, no one knows who built it or when. It's like the place just arose out of the mists of time, or something—the reason they call it the Old Course is because by the time people were writing things down about it, it had already been there for so long that people just accepted its existence as a fact of life.

When I was in high school, there was a spot down by the river called "the Land" where kids would go to party on weekends. It was a secret to everyone but high schoolers (and the cops, who despite never coming down there always seemed to camp out on nearby roads, waiting for drunk drivers). Over time, Jeeps and muddied sneakers and dragged coolers and kegs created walking trails down there. Someone brought in a bench or two, some ashtrays, maybe even a really gross trash can, and after a few generations of teens had built it up for the common pursuit of drinking six Bud Lights and then throwing up, the Land eventually became something of an unofficial public park. That's a good way to think about how St. Andrews came into being: collectively created over time, its exact design determined by the wisdom of the crowd. At some point, someone probably vomited there, too.

It's important to realize that golf's creation myth is really an inflection point in a larger, iterative process, one that dates back hundreds of years before the Old Course at St. Andrews came about and is still playing out today. Basically, people have been using sticks to hit ball-like things pretty much forever, and at some point, someone arbitrarily decided to look at this historical continuity of golf-like games and proclaimed that the sport became "golf" at the moment when Scottish people adapted them to the linksland environment and introduced the concept of aiming your ball at a hole in the ground.

But what was golf before golf? And when did golf become real golf? Some people have claimed the game has its roots in ancient Rome or even ancient Egypt. But when I say "some people," I specifically mean "some people on the internet," and the games they cite are basically games where people used a stick to hit a thing at another thing, but in a field hockey kind of way. Does that count as a super-early form of golf? I don't know. Maybe? Probably not? Whatever—it's fine either way.

To me, the strongest case to be made is that golf originated in China as a game called *chui wan*, which, when given the most literal translation possible, comes out as "ball stick." Ball stick, aka *chui wan*, is what happens when you combine polo, which the Chinese began playing in the seventh century as a way to help sharpen the equestrian skills of its military cavalry, with the Song dynasty's focus around AD 1000 on the moral teachings of Confucius.

Basically, at some point, Chinese peasants figured out they could play polo without riding horses, which gets us down on the ground hitting a ball with a club. Still, the purpose of polo with or without a horse was to help soldiers learn to move in formation and work together on the battlefield, so in order to make the jump to golf, someone was going to have to take fighting out of the equation. Fast-forward to AD 960, when, after decades of violent political upheaval throughout the country, a general named Zhao Kuangyin supposedly got drunk in his tent one night and woke up to his troops declaring him the new emperor. As Emperor Taizu, through a combination of diplomacy and military might, he quickly consolidated all the warlord-led territories throughout the region into a larger, relatively peaceful kingdom and established what became known as the Song dynasty. These folks ushered in a truly mind-boggling number of cool things, including paper money, gunpowder, a form of the printing press, magnetic compasses, and water-powered mechanical clocks. Part of what drove this new era of Chinese enlightenment was a tweaked spin on Confucian philosophy, which emphasized cultivating self-discipline, self-knowledge, good manners, and good character. In other words, Confucius didn't want you to play field hockey against somebody else—he wanted you to find the strength within to play golf against yourself.

The basic setup of *chui wan*, according to the 1282 book *Wan Jing*, was that you'd dig some holes in the ground, stick some flags in them, and hit walnut-size balls at them with a bamboo stick. (Archaeologists have actually recovered old *chui wan* balls that, like a modern Titleist, have little dimples carved into their covers to promote spin and hang time once the ball's in the air.) Like modern golf, the point was to get the ball into the hole in the fewest number of strokes, but because these people were working backward from polo, *chui wan* was a team game. It had a weird scoring system, and there were only three clubs. The players kept their own score, and winning teams weren't supposed to be a bunch of jerks to the losers. In the world of *chui wan*, everyone was a winner, because the true goal of the game was to hang out and have fun in nature.

So, now we're up to the Middle Ages, and we've got proto-golf in China. How does it get to the rest of Europe? Chinese scholars—a few of whom it should be noted, are *really* invested in playing up the *chui wan*–golf connection—have suggested that during the thirteenth or fourteenth century, the game casually slipped through the continental borders as a natural side effect of the greater cross-cultural exchange that was happening between Europe and Asia up until a little after the time the Black Death hit, around 1350. Thanks to merchants, missionaries, and the odd Mongol invasion, their thinking goes, China passed along gunpowder, printing, and the compass to Europe, so why couldn't they have passed along golf, too?

If *chui wan* made the journey from China to Europe (and I'm not a historian, so I'm simply saying that this *could* have happened), then the game spent a few years going off in a bunch of different directions before it became golf in Scotland. From at least 1270, there was a game called *choule* or *crosse* in France that was kind of like a mix of croquet and golf, while in Italy, Leonardo da Vinci wrote in 1492 about people playing a game that we'd later call "Pall Mall," which was somewhat akin to mini-golf but with fighting. The closest link between golf and not-golf comes from the Netherlands, where people were really into a game called *het kolven* or *colf* starting around the 1300s. The goal was to use a stick to hit a ball at a target, and the winner was whoever got there in the fewest number of strokes. Unlike modern golf, people played colf in the streets or on frozen lakes and did so in pretty close quarters, and they were totally fine hitting someone else's ball if it was in the way of their own. Given that there weren't any established rules to the game other than "drink heavily while playing colf," it's not exactly surprising that, similarly to Pall Mall, many colf sessions devolved into massive brawls.

At some point, colf split in two. In the Netherlands, it was co-opted by wealthy merchants and turned into a game called *kolf*, which was kind of like shuffleboard-meets-curling-meets-golf and was played in high-class drinking halls. Participants liked to wear fancy clothes while they played, and fighting was strongly discouraged. Boooooooooooo!

Meanwhile, during the 1400s, colf migrated over to Scotland's eastern coast, where it moved from the streets to the links, the local term for the grassy areas between the sea and farmable land, and became golf. Despite the change in venue, the improvised rules and air of boozy pugilism carried over. Victories might be determined not by who reached the target in the fewest number of strokes, but by which player got there first. If the term "blue-collar" had existed back then, golf would have been a blue-collar sport.

Once the Industrial Revolution hit Scotland, though, things changed. Out of the nation's peat bogs rose a new class of rich commoners, those who'd had the good sense to own the factories and mills that were transforming Europe, as opposed to those suckers who'd been conscripted by the forces of capital to work in them. But because of a quirk in Scotland's system of land rights, members of this freshly affluent social group couldn't buy or marry their way into the nobility. This must have been a bummer. Personally, I wouldn't start a yarn factory if I didn't think I'd get some sort of fancy title out of the deal. Then again, it was a different time, so maybe these people went into their industrial endeavors with clear eyes and full hearts. Regardless, members of this new "between" class wanted a way to differentiate themselves from the rabble out of which they rose, and golf, the beloved folk pastime of the Scottish seaside, proved to be just the ticket.

These folks formed clubs, which instituted rules requiring players to adhere to specific codes of dress and conduct, charged membership fees, and transformed golf from this weird product of drunken improvisation into a fully regulated sport. Perhaps most importantly for the evolution of the game, these clubs bought patches of land and erected permanent courses upon them, turning spaces that were once public and communal into ones that were private and exclusive. I guess if you can't live in a castle, the next best thing is to form a club with all your friends, make up a bunch of arcane, boring rules, and tell all the poor people they're not cool enough to join. To me, it all seems very reminiscent of middle school.

The first golf club that left us written proof of its existence was called the Honourable Company of Edinburgh Golfers, which dates back to at least 1744, the year when, under an earlier name, it published a list of thirteen rules for an upcoming tournament. I will now take the liberty of quoting some of the more goofily written ones:

> *5. If your Ball comes along watter, or any topy filth, you are at liberty to take out your Ball & bringing it behind the hazard and Teeing it, you may play it with any Club and allow your Adversary a Stroke for so getting out your Ball.*
> *8. If you should lose your Ball, by it's being taken up, or any other way, you are to go back to the Spot, where you struct last, & drop another Ball, And allow your adversary a Stroke for the misfortune.*
> *10. If a Ball be stop'd by any Person, Horse, Dog, or anything else, The Ball so stop'd must be play'd where it lyes.*

Overall, the game that the HCEG sketched out more or less resembles golf as we know it today. You counted your strokes, took penalties when necessary, and in all other situations, played your ball wherever it landed (even if it ricocheted off a horse). The tournament was won by a guy named John Rattray, who was awarded a silver club and got to be known as the captain of all golf for the entire year. The next year, Rattray was sentenced to death for taking part in an uprising against the king, only for one of his golf buddies to pull some strings with the local duke and have the execution called off, which marks the first time in recorded history that a friendship seeded on the golf course blossomed into full-on nepotism.

There's a bit of confusion over whether Rattray, whose signature was present at the bottom of the rules, wrote them himself, or simply signed them because he'd just won and was endorsing them as Captain Golf. But if the guy who wrote the rules won the game, it seems like he probably cheated. Regardless, the rules were quickly adopted by other clubs throughout Scotland and England, and that's . . . sort of how we got golf.

• • •

When I was a kid, I never thought about how the things around me got there. Buildings, towns, systems, and concepts were older than me, and therefore it seemed easier to just accept them as they were and have that be that. Golf was this green monolith, its customs and formats seemingly fixed. But when I dug a little deeper, I began to realize that golf is constantly evolving, and that it's the people who play it who drive those changes. For proof, look no further than the golf tee, the etymology of which the golf historian Neil Laird suggests is derived from the Dutch word *tuitje*, meaning "little cone." Originally, golfers would carry pouches of sand around to create a mound off of which they'd hit their ball, which was obviously inconvenient and in no way ideal (while elevating the ball gives you more accuracy because of a lack of impediments, sand itself is an impediment—it slows clubhead speed down, thereby robbing you of distance). It wasn't until 1899 that a Black dentist named George Grant, the son of escaped enslaved people, realized that since the job of a tee was to elevate the ball while it rested on a small indentation, you could replicate the indentation in a piece of wood, and it'd be sturdier than sand yet thin enough to not slow down a swing.

Generally, the concept that we term "innovation" occurs when a bunch of people all over the place are all fumbling toward different versions of the same thing, and at some point, someone does something seemingly random that propels a specific version of the thing to break through. Henry Ford introduced the conveyor belt to the already-happening phenomenon of the assembly line, and so his name is synonymous with mass production, Mark Zuckerberg decided that social networks should be based around people we already know, and that's why we're all on Facebook, and the people of the Lowlands in Scotland made the most lasting version of a game that had happened all over the place, so they get credit for creating golf.

But as the world changes, so do the stories we tell about it. Over the past few decades, China as a whole has become a massive player on the global stage, and its historians understandably want to assert a view of the past that centralizes their country in the conversation. Telling your history is a way of saying that you matter. And frankly, there's absolutely no way of knowing who invented golf. But *chui wan*'s existence, and the fact that it's in this conversation, speaks to the universal nature of creativity. All over the world, since time immemorial, humans have enjoyed hitting a little ball with a big stick, and that impulse transcends class or social standing.

Ultimately, the history of golf is one of how ideas and concepts spread, as well as what we in the present do with the fragments of evidence that our ancestors left behind. Golf wasn't a massive political or social movement, nor was it some magnificent invention that helped usher in our modern age. It was just a thing that regular people did for fun when they weren't worried about working or dying. There's a term, "NARP—Not a Real Person," that characters in the TV show *Succession* use to refer to the unwashed, unseen masses, and even though no one has ever said this out loud in the real world, it's a concept that can help us understand why the history of golf is so hard to nail down. For centuries, the people who knew how to read and write—and *whose writing people thought to preserve*—worked in the royal court or the church. We get a textual record of the stuff that happened around kings, military generals, and high-up church officials, but nobody thought that people in the future would want to know about the NARPs, even those who made major contributions to the world. For them, we're left with a shard of engraved pottery, an unearthed piece of iron found in a long-gone village, a body found in a peat bog whose scars ache to tell its story.

Trying to trace the objective history of golf by correctly interpreting the open-ended evidence that we have is, in a way, maddening. But that impossibility can also be utterly liberating. Golf is ancient, yet unburdened by the specificity of events, and we're free to sift through the jumbled pieces that others have gone over a thousand times before, assembling the stories that help the game make sense for us. A field is never just a field, and the past is never just the past. Some Scottish farmers taught me that. I think one of them made golf clubs.

Chapter Three

HOW GOLF KEEPS ME HONEST

ONE OF THE reasons they say golf is good for kids is that it teaches them math skills. You understand addition through totaling up your score, figure out how to translate numbers on a page into real-life space through tracking yardages and reading the slope of a green, and learn personal finance through calculating how much money your parents would need to make every year in order to become members at the country club where you just played a junior golf tournament. Growing up, I was never that good at the math part of golf, which is why, when I moved out of my parents' house for the second time at twenty-seven, I decided against buying a three-bedroom house close to downtown Durham that had a $750 monthly mortgage and instead paid $800 a month to rent a garage near the highway.

I mean, it was a pretty nice garage. The lady whose house it was next to had sealed up the garage door part of it, put in one of those space-age air conditioners that exist only in guesthouses, and reversed the front door's hinges so her tenants could have a clear path to the stairs that led to the attic, which was now a bedroom.

It wasn't up to code, but what *is* code, anyway? Upstairs, there was a bed, a cedar chest, a small skylight, an even smaller window, and a chair with the legs cut off, resting directly upon unsteady, carpet-covered floorboards. Even though my landlord had raised the ceiling so high that I could feel the rain hit the roof when I lay in bed, it was still fundamentally an attic, and I couldn't really stand all the way up in it. Downstairs, there was a fridge, a hot plate, a couch, a TV, and a dining room table that I immediately repurposed as a desk. The bathroom, which had a sliding door and no lock, and all the closets were also downstairs, and now that I think about it, I should have used the upstairs as the living room and the downstairs as a combination kitchen-bedroom.

I chose the garage because it seemed like a good deal. It was my first time living fully on my own, no roommates and no house rules, and seeing as I felt like a baby bird who'd just pecked out of its egg, anything seemed like a good deal—the house I'd almost bought also seemed like a good, but way more complicated, deal, so I went with the good deal that was less of a commitment.

I have no idea if twenty-seven is late or early or normal to start living by yourself, but that seemed like a good deal, too. Most people I know go out into the world, live with roommates until they get into a serious relationship, then move in with that person, and if they break up, they go back to the roommates. The older they get, the fewer roommates they have, until they wake up one day and realize they're too rich or old or weird to live with anyone. I was none of those things. Or at least I definitely wasn't rich, I probably wasn't old, and regardless of the actual evidence, I'd always told myself I was only weird in a fun, non-alienating way. And besides, parents are great and all, but they're terrible roommates.

My place was disgusting. It was me and Nora, the dog. The thing they don't tell you about dogs is that they're like two-year-olds. And they have about the same level of control over their bodily functions as a two-year-old. I once left the garage to play eighteen holes and came back to discover that the dog had left diarrhea all over the carpet, the couch, my records, and the bathroom floor. I got the poop off the dog and the floors and the couch, but everything smelled slightly like it should not have smelled. In time, it began to feel as if the walls were closing in on me, but that was just an optical illusion caused by the accumulation of clothes, books, records, spare irons and woods and putters sourced from thrift stores, handwritten drafts and lists, and an unopened Nintendo Wii my parents foisted upon me, as well as generalized, unsorted clutter. I'm one of those people who, once I put something somewhere, that's the new place that that thing lives, be it a cup on a table, a jacket on the couch, or a broken typewriter I appointed as a decorative flourish next to the upstairs chair.

To be fair to myself, I didn't spend *that* much time there. At least one week out of every month, I'd drop the dog off with my parents and take an airplane up to New York to see my girlfriend and try to schedule a meeting with an editor so I could write off the trip on my taxes. When I was home, I played lots of golf, but I didn't golf as much as I wrote, because golf and plane tickets and coffee cost money. OK, I guess I spent a good bit of time there. But I kept the floor around the desk clear, and I spilled water on my notes only once, and only a few of them formed an ad hoc papier-mâché surface on the desk itself, and I managed to razor it off when I moved out.

I had so many questions I'd never thought about before. Which bills did I have to pay on time, and which ones could I ignore for a while? When was I supposed to sleep? When was I supposed to work? When was I supposed to hang out? When we're alone, there's a danger of all structure breaking down, causing us to devolve into a state of madness. Some nights, I wouldn't start writing until midnight, and some days, I wouldn't wake up until early afternoon. Other days, I'd be filling in for my editor at a weed website owned by Snoop Dogg, and I'd wake up at eight in the morning. Some days, I remembered I had a coffee maker and a fridge and bread and pasta and fresh vegetables and salad dressing, while other days, I bought four bacon, egg, and cheese biscuits and grazed upon them throughout the day. We establish baselines in life, and they have a sneaky way of readjusting themselves when we've looked away for too long. Then something happens and we take a step back, ask ourselves if this is how we really are, and suddenly those baselines jump back up again. Growing up is what happens when we aspire, in these moments, to stay on the right side of socialization.

Golf is a great way to learn to do things for yourself. Even when you're playing with other people, you're playing only *against* yourself, keeping your own score and holding yourself accountable to a set of rules that it is your own responsibility to internalize. If you break those rules, no one else is going to penalize or punish you. Perhaps they will judge you silently, but never as harshly as they are judging you silently on the golf course of your imagination. Most of the time, the only punishment for doing something wrong is the guilt that we impose upon ourselves. That guilt can be good, so long as we sit with it, ponder it, allowing ourselves to process and learn from it so that we may become a little bit better next time. I just looked up that house I almost bought, by the way—it's tripled in value in five years. It's fine. Nobody knows what's going to happen until it does.

Since their creation, the rules of golf have ballooned from thirteen precepts scrawled onto a single handwritten page to a series of twenty-four edicts, each with official interpretations, terminology, and technicalities, available in a 592-page printed edition as well as a free app, published by the United States Golf Association (USGA), that takes up 67.4 megabytes of space on a smartphone. That's bigger than the apps for the *New York Times*'s crossword puzzle, HBO Max's streaming player, or the download of Zoom's videoconferencing software.

As time has gone on, the rules have gotten more detailed and complex in ways that mostly don't matter, but which occasionally have drastic effects on the game. This happens because social mores and technology change over time, and if golf doesn't change with them, then it runs the risk of seeming even more archaic than it already does. For a while in the mid- to late 2000s, for example, club makers realized that if they made drivers and fairway woods with square heads, it would be easier for average golfers to make the ball go straight. This has something to do with how a square head shape affects a club's moment of inertia, which is a physics concept I don't fully understand, because the last time I took the subject was my senior year of high school, and I skipped it a lot. The point, though, is that only a couple of years after this technological advancement, these clubs became illegal to use in competition. Just as we must regulate AI before it enslaves humanity, we must prevent square-headed drivers from making bad golfers think they're better than they actually are.

When the rules were updated in 2019, meanwhile, the powers that be decided that, after decades of requiring players to take the flag stick out of the hole when they putted or else suffer a penalty stroke, it's now fine to leave it in. It's not a huge change in the grand scheme of things, but golfers have spent their lives taking the pin out. Was it all for naught? No, because we all knew it was stupid, and now the rules have adapted in an attempt to correct that stupidity.

As a work of literature, *The Rules of Golf* is the perfect combination of boring and insane. When playing golf by the book, you can be penalized for things like conspiracy to commit rule breaking, asking the wrong question, building your own golf club during a round, or even listening to music that is of the same tempo as your golf swing. There are also sections of the rule book establishing how one should treat things like fruit ("Fruit that is detached from its tree or bush is a loose impediment, even if the fruit is from a bush or tree not found on the course," we learn, but "when being carried by a player, it is his or her equipment") and human saliva (which, depending on the preference of the player, "may be treated as either temporary water or a loose impediment"). It tells us that we can't place a bottle of water on certain parts of the green that might give you an unnatural understanding of its slope, and, mysteriously, it makes it clear that there's a difference between a tree and a wooden bench. You're allowed to move things like spiderwebs, sticks, stones, snow, worms, anthills, dead animals, and animal poop if they're close enough to your ball that they interfere with your ability to swing, stand, or hit the ball. Human poop is not discussed within the rules, but I guess you'd be allowed to relocate your ball under Rule 24, which provides relief from "man-made obstructions." Though if we consider human poop natural once it's on the ground, that goes into some thorny philosophical territory as to the true nature of humanity—are we mere beasts, or do we serve a higher calling? For the purposes of not having to inhale the stench of manure while trying to hit my four-iron, I'm going with the former.

The rules get pretty metaphysical, too. There's an entire section dedicated to "natural forces," which are defined this way: "The effects of nature such as wind, water, or when something happens for no apparent reason because of the effects of gravity." What is reason? What do we allow ourselves to see, and what do we intentionally blind ourselves to? Is it a good idea to smoke weed while you play golf? There are no answers here, only more questions.

If you read the rules in their entirety, a few themes tend to jump out: They value fairness and honesty, as well as earning your score through skill and athleticism rather than through gimmicks or artificial manipulation. And in fact, the first rule of golf is that you have to play by the rules. Rule 1 defines the rules of golf as Rules 1–24 of *The Rules of Golf* and states that "players are responsible for applying the Rules to themselves." The idea that people can and should be trusted to do the right thing even when no one's watching is kind of magical, almost utopian. If we lived in a world in which the Constitution existed in a permanent state of revision, evolving based on the needs of our society at any given moment, and every law had a rational justification rooted in fairness and honesty for everyone, we would live in a police-free paradise where we all had flying cars and they were constantly playing disco music. Just some food for thought.

• • •

Like nearly every golfer, I have a hard time following the rules. It's not that I don't care or that I cheat per se, it's just that there are a lot of them and most of them are meant for tournaments played on fancy courses whose every blade of grass is trimmed with intentionality and not a single speck of pine straw meanders past the tree line.

When you're playing a normal round on a normal golf course, meanwhile, there are higher loyalties to consider, and the concept of "playing it as it lies" becomes a luxury that few of us can afford. There are divots in the fairway whose infinitesimal depression in the earth throws a bucket of variables into the equation that you really shouldn't be dealing with. Ball marks on the green, relics of one careless golfer after another who couldn't be bothered to fix the little depression their approach shot has left, a true tragedy of the commons that leaves the putting area looking like the surface of the moon. Inexplicable patches of hard, red clay dirt where there should be grass, posing a risk to the life of the clubs and the structural integrity of the limbs belonging to those bullheaded enough to try to hit off them. People behind you who are going to get very annoyed if you spend your allotted minutes searching for an errant Titleist when they'd very much like to tee off at the exact spot you left your golf bag.

And so we have the unwritten rules of golf, which are instituted in the same spirit as the official ones, even when the former sometimes fly in the face of the latter. You move the ball when it's in a bad lie, because the economy isn't good enough for your local course to fix the fairways. You drop a ball when you've lost your first one rather than playing a provisional, because the mental pressure of trying to play fast when you've got drunk people behind you is too high for most of us. Those two shots out of the sand magically become one, because life is hard and your playing partner understands this and sometimes they're willing to look the other way.

But then there are further indulgences, things as decadent as waking up at noon and proceeding to smoke weed with your roommate until you're both high enough to eat a whole pizza each. In the context of golf, this means hitting a poor shot, dropping another ball and hitting it, then pretending your first ball never existed—aka the much-frowned-upon but all-too-common mulligan.

For me, this plays out in the following way:

1. I swing poorly, usually due to the tempo of my swing being off, and hook my ball into an unplayable abyss.
2. Instead of trudging up there, retrieving my ball, taking the penalty stroke (or two, depending on the circumstances), and continuing with the knowledge that I probably won't make par, I reject reality, insist that my first shot never happened, and, flush with frustration, take a mulligan and drop another ball.
3. My second shot is marginally less crappy than my first, and I end up scoring just as badly, if not worse, as I would have if I'd just taken my medicine. Shaken, I continue to struggle through the rest of the round.

OR:

3A. My second shot turns out great and I end up with a par that, in my soul, I know is unearned. Wracked with guilt, my subconscious blows up the rest of my round in an act of righteous self-sabotage.

Regardless of knowing that this is the inevitable outcome, the temptation to take a do-over in the form of a mulligan is always there. One of the great tragedies of life is that we cannot take back what we have already put into the world. But golf, with its focus on self-regulation without outside oversight, creates the ideal conditions to bend the rules in the hope of changing our fate. It's instructive that this rarely works out. Even if I artificially engineer a better result in the short term, soon enough the contradictions pile up and overload my brain. When I hit a bad shot and try to move forward from there, I'm accepting the world as it exists. I resolve the issue, closing the loop so that I have a chance to do better next time. Taking a mulligan offers no such relief, only the illusion of the quick fix.

There is no such thing as perfect golf, only avoiding error, mitigating bad outcomes when they occur so that we end up with no worse than a bogey, and capitalizing on the occasional birdie opportunity that arises out of an ever-shifting triangulation of skill and luck. Mulligans deny this basic truth of the game and instead scream, "I want perfect, and I want it now!" But really, this type of thinking is just buying into some weird sense of false pride.

Intuitively, I know that the only way to make the number of errors per round trend downward and the number of birdie opportunities trend upward is to embrace those very same errors. A pretty good first shot doesn't lead to a second shot so good that it leaves you with a makeable birdie putt on its own. You've got to burst through a wall of self-imposed pressure in order to get there. And the best way to train yourself to manage that pressure is to face it head-on, over and over again. Soon enough, you realize that one lousy shot isn't that big of a deal; it's just a thing that happens. Once you understand that it's possible—normal, even—to follow a bad shot with a good one, stringing a few of them together to nab a birdie begins to feel a whole lot easier, because each hole no longer feels like walking a tightrope with no room for error. The lights come on, and we see that the tightrope has been hovering three inches off the ground the entire time.

I believe all of this wholeheartedly, yet I still find myself taking extra shots, often ending up halfway through a swing before my brain even processes what my body's gone ahead and done. I do this because of the natural human instinct to avoid pain, both mental and physical, real and perceived. We put off doing the laundry, taking our cars to get an oil change, and paying our bills, not because they're actually difficult, but because they're not fun. No matter how much we try to push them out of our mind, the knowledge that they must be done is still there, nagging at us. *This is the last one today*, I tell myself as I set a second ball down, *this is bad and stupid, but I've got twelve more holes to do it right*. But it's never the last one, and suddenly they've shut the water off in my apartment because I couldn't be bothered to pay the bill or even put my account on auto-pay.

For those of us with the privilege of knowing more or less where we'll land if we fall, this mentality, I think, is vestigial, a holdover from humanity's early days when there were *actual* things to worry about. Cutting your hand on a rock could very well have led to infection and then death. The rustle in those tall reeds next to the lake might have just been the wind, or maybe it meant there was a big crocodile lying in wait to eat you. Eat the wrong plant or animal, meanwhile, and you'd catch a disease and die. Even up until a few decades ago, there were a number of shockingly easy ways to die, and so fear and avoidance were probably great survival tools. But this is golf or modern adulthood, or both, we're talking about here. As much as our long-held instincts might argue otherwise, there's nothing truly painful about opening our banking app so that we can check our balance and pay down our credit card, or punching the second shot of the hole out into the fairway and setting ourselves up for an easy bogey.

In a court case, there are so many laws, statutes, and precedents on the books that a good lawyer can select the specific ones most favorable to the client and build an argument from there. We see this most flagrantly in the tax world, where large companies have not only America's tax laws but those of the entire world to select from, which allows a company like, say, Apple to set up holding companies in Ireland and therefore manage to pay next to nothing in taxes in any country. The rules of golf are sort of the opposite of that. Golfers have no lawyers, only themselves, and it's rare that they are presented with a situation in which the more favorable outcome applies. If your ball lands in a depression on the green that you then fix so that you can place your ball for putting and it happens to roll into the hole, you don't get to count it as going in through an act of God, like a clause in an insurance contract. If you lose or break a club while playing, you can't borrow another one, or else it's a two-stroke penalty on the first two holes on which you use that club (but unlike the rolling-ball rule, if a club breaks and it isn't your fault, you *can* replace it). Perhaps most maddeningly, you can move your ball if it lands in a hole made by an animal, but not when it lands in an animal's footprint, which seems counterintuitive. If your ball's stuck in a rabbit hole, you definitely risk getting your hand nipped by the rabbit who owns that hole. Might be best to change the rule so that you can leave it and take a free drop.

However, this doesn't mean that the entire game is meant to punish you or make it so that you can't win if you suck. This is where the concept of handicaps come in, the philosophy of which I'll explain with my favorite myth. It's from *Book of the Hopi*, Frank Waters's transcriptions of Hopi legends told to him by tribe elders, and it goes like this: A young woman in a village proposes marriage to a boy from the Coyote Clan, but another boy, from the Swallow Clan, had nearly won the girl's heart (all the village boys came to talk to her through her window while she shucked corn, and she eliminated her suitors one by one until she wanted to talk only to the boy from the Coyote Clan while shucking), and now the Swallow Clan has proposed that the two boys race. They'll run through a forest and back to the village, where a pair of obsidian knives are waiting in the ground. Whoever comes back first gets to use the knife to chop the other kid's head off, and then he can also marry the young woman. I know this is gruesome, but bear with me.

The boys start the race, with Coyote Boy—the one we're rooting for, remember—taking an initial lead, only to be passed by Swallow Boy because he used magic to turn himself into a bird. This is obviously not ideal if you're Coyote Boy, so he takes a break to commune with the spirits of his Coyote brethren, who use *their* magical powers to make it rain so hard that Swallow Boy, who has transformed himself into a literal swallow, can no longer fly in the storm. They then help Coyote Boy create a kind of hovercraft out of a gourd and some string so that he can catch up to Swallow Boy. Once the competitors are dead even (I'm foreshadowing by using the word "dead"), the Coyote Clan mandates that the suitors have to finish the race without any magical aids. So they both run like hell toward the village, and as they approach the finish line, Coyote Boy makes a mad dive ahead of Swallow Boy, doing a *Mission: Impossible*–style combat roll in which he grabs his knife and chops Swallow Boy's head off in one swift, fluid motion. Coyote Boy and the young woman proceed with their wedding, the Swallow Clan gets ejected from the village, and everyone who doesn't have a name including the word "Swallow" lives happily ever after.

I love this story for a lot of reasons—the twists! the divine intervention! the punishment for disrupting the matriarchal nature of society being decapitation!—but also because it shows that the attitude driving the handicap system is a universal one. Handicaps are basically legal cheating—they represent the number of strokes that, based on your performance over a series of past rounds, you're allowed to take off your score while competing or betting with someone else. If I'm a 13 handicap and I'm playing golf with a friend who's an 8 handicap, that means that if I shoot an 86 against his 82, I still win, because 86 minus 13 is 73, and 82 minus 8 is 74.

Of course, the handicap system is only as useful as the scores you use to calculate it. Ill-gotten scores will make your handicap lower than it should be, yielding less of an advantage when you actually need it. I've been guilty of doing this, due to vanity or insecurity or both. Just as the stock market exists to make the big number go up, we play golf to make the small number go down, and there's always the temptation to make it go down faster than it should. That's the ultimate lesson conveyed by that Hopi legend, too. Both Coyote Boy and Swallow Boy cheated in the race, but when they were courting the young woman, she chose Coyote Boy; rather than respecting her decision like he should have, Swallow

Boy declared a mulligan and made the race happen. Coyote Boy earned his handicap (his proto-hovercraft made out of a gourd) through dedication and honesty, so it's only natural that he should win the race and that Swallow Boy must die an excruciatingly painful death in front of all his loved ones.

Maintaining a handicap is an exercise in monastic self-discipline. The scores I am most ashamed of are the ones that will ultimately save me when it comes time to put that handicap to good use. When I first started tracking mine, I reported only the good scores I notched, and the fact that I had a handicap that suggested I was a stronger player than I truly was felt more valuable than having something that was, shall we say, a tad more realistic. What was once a handicap of 9 grew closer to 15. When I posted a round full of lost balls, duck hooks, and three-putts, the fact that in the long run it might help me win ten bucks off my friend Charlie (handicap of 7, intimidatingly long driver) someday made it hurt that much less.

But there are golfers who take this mentality too far in the other direction, artificially inflating their handicaps in order to hustle some mark. This is especially prevalent in amateur tournaments, where a good golfer with a bad handicap can run away with the whole thing. Imagine if Coyote Boy had pretended to break his leg at the beginning of the race and had used that as an excuse to stay in his gourd hovercraft all the way to the finish line. Handicaps require good faith.

I first read that Hopi story a few years ago while sitting in the Rothko Chapel in Houston, during a cross-country road trip with my friend Kyle. It's a dimly lit, octagonal room, each wall covered by a dark-hued canvas by the late painter Mark Rothko. Inside, you can sit, stand, lie down, meander around the floor, whatever you'd like to do, really, as long as you're doing it silently. I personally know very little about art, so I couldn't tell you what differentiates the towering, color-block paintings inside from ones that anyone else could make, at least on a technical level. The point is not necessarily to consider the canvases themselves, but instead to bask in the aura of the room, allowing this space of reverence, so open to interpretation, to carry you where it may. In that spirit, the chapel's custodians have a rack of literature from dozens of faiths and traditions near the entrance, from which visitors are encouraged to pick a book at random to read inside. If you give yourself over to the physical and emotional confines of the space, you tend to give yourself over to something larger than yourself. The canvases begin to suck light in, and soon enough they've sucked you in, too, transporting you to a new plane of being, upon which you are at peace. Sometimes, if you follow the rules of the room, you gain an understanding of why they're there in the first place.

I have an unfortunate habit of occasionally slipping into a state of quiet, contemplative despair. I dwell on mistakes I've made in the past as if they somehow demean my present or hobble my future. Sometimes, it's as minor as viewing a hangover as a moral failing rather than a natural consequence of drinking too much at a friend's house the night before, ignoring the fact that I took a cab home rather than put others at risk by driving drunk. Other times, I think back to when I was in college, more interested in having fun and playing dusty rap records in the middle of the night at my college radio station than I was in studying, and I start to wonder if my life would have turned out differently if I'd just applied myself and tried to go to grad school or something. If I'd just become an academic instead of a writer, I tell myself, I would have found a purpose. Structure. Stability. In this unexpressed alternate life, I am never depressed. "But I didn't do those things," my negative self says, "and that's somehow why I ended up having a nervous breakdown."

Thinking this way, of course, is both absurd and unhelpful. I took the shots I took, some turned out well and some didn't, and it doesn't matter either way because I'm here. In golf (if you follow the rules), you cannot change your score or take back a shot. But that's OK, because in time you learn that basing your enjoyment of the game off the numbers you write down on the scorecard is a recipe for hating golf, because those numbers will never be low enough. Understanding this is liberating. You're just a passenger on this big train that's chugging along, and we can't control what's in the past any more than we can control what's out the window. You can move around in the train, grab a snack in the dining car, or try to sneak into first class, but the rest is just scenery. By embracing agency over the present, we allow ourselves to place the things we can't control in perspective.

As I got more zealous about not taking mulligans, my scores started going up, but I felt better about saying them out loud. They were mine, even the ones that stank. There's quiet dignity in stinking, I think—especially when it's on our own terms.

Chapter Four

HOW GOLF TAUGHT ME TO SLOW DOWN

THE INTERNET IS bad. It's scary, everyone on it is insane, and even the people there who aren't criminals are still trying to scam you. I know this well, because once upon a time, I worked on the internet and also spent my free time talking with friends I'd made over the internet about what was happening on it. I was employed by a very cool music website owned by a very cool company in Brooklyn, and my coworkers and I all got discounts at a bunch of the stores and restaurants within a two-mile radius of our office, which was really important because we were, as a general rule, paid salaries that were slightly below the New York City poverty threshold. The trick that this company figured out is that if you hire twenty-three-year-olds and work them seventy hours a week while paying them next to nothing, they'll be really excited about it as long as you convince them that their job makes them culturally influential, or at least automatically interesting at parties. Almost no one I worked with had a degree in journalism or any training whatsoever, so we mostly just made up the rules as we went along.

I went to my interview there stoned; when I announced this to my boss-to-be, he laughed and offered me the gig on the spot.

It was my job to write and edit articles, mainly about rap music, that lots of people would click on. Clicks translated to readers and page views, which translated to advertisers giving my employer money, which translated to my coworkers and me keeping our jobs. The way our bosses determined the "growth" of our "audience" was through the self-explanatory metric of "unique viewers," which was in spirit supposed to be the number of reliable readers we had, but we always suspected that lots of different people were just reading one of our articles once before promptly forgetting that our site existed. Regardless, we had a subscription to a service called Chartbeat, which would tell us how many people were on which parts of our website at any given time; through obsessively checking it, we began to figure out some basic heuristics of what worked on the internet.

First, the headlines were really important. They needed to be descriptive, hyperbolic, and tantalizing, yet still short enough to fit into a Tweet and never follow a set formula. Nouns, especially proper nouns, were good (except if readers had never heard of the person we were writing about), as were questions and, conversely, firmly declarative statements. This was confusing and contradictory, but we did our best, and ended up with headlines like "Kanye West Just Unleashed a Gift to Foot Fetishists Everywhere," "Last Night a Limp Bizkit Concert Converted Me to the Church of Nu-Metal," and "What the Fuck Is Going On with This Satan-Worshiping Teen Rapper's Face Tattoo?" It didn't really matter to our boss's bosses if people actually read the articles, which was fine with us because it meant we could write crazy stuff when we wanted to, or we could just not try at all and write barely anything.

Ironically, though, we also discovered that sometimes people seemed to want to read the articles, or at least the first couple of paragraphs of them. So right at the beginning of whatever you wrote, you had to say what your point was, because hopefully people would read a little bit of it and decide to share it on social media because it reinforced some sort of uncomplicated, strong feeling they had about the world. If we were super-complimentary about a musician (or if we'd worked out a deal with their publicist beforehand), they might share our article on their Facebook page, lending us the eyeballs of their adoring fans and making the Chartbeat numbers go up. If you were ruthlessly mean about something and packed your article with every one-liner and pithy put-down you could think of, you'd be inundated with clicks and shares, both from people egging on your mean-spirited jokes and those who'd fallen for the ruse and were spreading your article out of this Pavlovian rage response, which entailed their getting specifically mad at you, the author of the article.

• • •

One great thing about the internet is that it has drastically reduced the cost of gathering information, both in terms of monetary cost and the time it takes to access that information. If I want to find out how many major championships Nicklaus won during his career, all I need to do is google "Jack Nicklaus majors," and his eighteen victories pop right up. But if it were 1989 and I wanted to figure it out, I might have to drive to the library and leaf through books, magazines, and news articles on microfilm in order to get that same information. Or I could go to the pro shop of my local golf course and ask a group of clubhouse rats who happened to be sitting on the patio drinking beer that same question, and watch as they argued among themselves: "Fifteen majors." "No, nineteen, or actually eighteen, because the '86 Masters shouldn't count because Greg Norman and Tom Kite probably let him win because he was a legend." "No! That counts double since he was so old and it should have been impossible!" At its best, the internet adds a dose of objectivity to our lives. Or, more darkly, maybe it just means we don't need to know anything anymore as long as we have access to a smartphone.

This has been great for everyday people who just want to confirm basic, objective facts about Jack Nicklaus. But it hasn't been very good for the news media, which used to specialize in gathering information, bundling it into a newspaper or magazine, and then selling it to people (and then selling those people to advertisers, which was key). But as the internet overtook the printed page as the main way people got their information, it made what newsrooms have always been great at doing worth a whole lot less.

When a story runs in a print publication, it's part of a greater whole—even if only a few people actually read what you've written, the story still adds value to the overall package the reader is getting. Back in the day—even up until the mid-2010s—a magazine might have had a celebrity on the cover and an accompanying profile inside its pages, but that would have sat alongside deeply reported investigative features, humor pieces, lists of weird factoids, buyers' guides, reviews, essays both highbrow and low, some regular columns, big-budget photo spreads, articles about emerging trends and ideas, and some letters to the editor that were occasionally made up. Every bit of the magazine existed in symbiosis with everything else, giving the reader a bunch of different options and therefore expanding the publication's hypothetical audience. All of this helped publishers charge top dollar for ads, maintain robust staffs, and pay freelance writers at a relative premium. It helped, too, that magazines operated from a place of information asymmetry when dealing with advertisers. They often grossly exaggerated their scope of influence by claiming that each issue of a publication had a "pass-along rate," meaning that multiple people were actually reading each copy, reinventing their readerships as "audiences" of people who maybe just flipped through a magazine without actually reading anything but still saw an ad or two. Often, the same publishers who benefited from these inflated or made-up metrics were also the primary funders of the firms that collected audience data. It was great.

But on the internet, every article stands alone; publications employ third-party software to measure traffic in real time, which keeps them honest; and the better a story is, the more likely everyone's just going to copy it. This is one of the many reasons the internet has driven ad prices on websites down. Another is human psychology. It seems like people believe that when they buy a physical copy of a publication, they're essentially paying for the paper it was printed on. This is only half true. Printing stuff costs money, yes, but so do the salaries of the people who put their experience, effort, and expertise into the stories that appear on that paper. This is way more abstract of a justification for charging money for something than "this is a stack of shiny paper we created," and so on the internet, people—and advertisers—expect stories to be free. By now, the people willing to pay to read even a great story, printed or not, have become a specialty market, not unlike those who buy music on vinyl.

In practical terms, the widespread decline of print marked a shift in the type of articles that most publications, including the one I worked for, ran. Rather than figuring out what was happening, they just started telling you what to think about it. Reporting is expensive; opinions are free. At twenty-three, I was dumb enough to think that this was a valuable service I was providing, and the fact that I didn't know much about anything seemed to give me the confidence to bless the world with my thoughts on a sometimes twice-daily basis.

On a strictly personal level, the death cycle of print media led to my getting punched in the head at two in the morning while standing outside a bar, by the friend of a rapper I'd recently written a mean article about. I'm going to tell you all about that, but first I need to tell you some more things about the internet.

Because of the way the internet works, I didn't need to be wise or experienced as much as I needed to play to the market. When you work as a writer on the internet, the internet is as much your boss as your actual boss is, because it's your actual boss's job to get a sense of whether or not the internet likes you. This can severely screw up your sense of self-worth, because even though you're supposed to be "leading the conversation" (this is a meaningless phrase, no matter what the people in marketing think), you're really performing for a potentially unlimited audience, and it doesn't matter whether they love you or are just there to throw tomatoes at you. In this context, especially if you're too young to realize this isn't normal, you sort of become like a dog whose main currency is attention. Positive attention is preferable, of course, but you'll take the negative over nothing every day of the week.

Though most of our traffic came from Facebook, the true fount of success in the online writing world, for me and an embarrassing number of my friends, was Twitter. If you wrote enough, even if it was bad, you'd build up your followers. One's Twitter followers were—and maybe still are, depending on when you're reading this—seen as a rough approximation of your audience, and therefore your influence, in this little digital world. My peers and I aspired to be planets in a solar system, our Twitter followers becoming bits of space junk that had once hurtled through the galaxy but were now trapped reliably within our gravitational pull. But each individual piece of space junk varied in size, and might have its own satellites in orbit around it, and we, the planets, may have been only moons around even larger planets, which themselves were merely pebbles when compared to the star at the center of it all. At times, this star has been Kanye West, Donald Trump, and Elon Musk.

Now, envision a million variants of this solar system existing in close proximity, with celestial bodies overlapping and intersecting and sharing custody of the space junk within their gravitational fields. Though many planets share common objects in their orbit, there will come a point, as you travel through this weird constellation of nonsense, where you stop seeing all the space rocks you're used to, and instead start encountering entirely new ones.

As my little planet got bigger and bigger and I dragged more and more nineteen-year-old space rocks into my orbit, never did I once stop and ask myself, "Is this healthy?" I was writing for the space rocks, and the space rocks were talking back, saying they liked it when I did some things and hated it when I did others. This cycle feels so good that you accept the low pay and the fact that by doing this, you've effectively tethered your self-esteem to a bunch of mercurial strangers with smartphones, and it continues to feel good even as you start to care less and less about the things that you're actually writing. I found myself in a death-spiraling feedback loop: People had decided that they liked it when I said snarky things about musicians whose work I disliked, and so I found myself doing it almost as a reflex when I couldn't think of something better to write about. Each time I wrote one of these unilateral pans, I tried to jam more hyperbolic invective into my prose, if only to keep myself from getting too bored. As cutting as I was, I typed them from a place of remove, usually assuming I was such a small fish that my targets wouldn't even see them, let alone read or react to them. And then a rapper I wrote a mean thing about sent a dude to punch me in the head.

Like most true stories these days, the actual particulars aren't that interesting. Basically, there was a rapper I had once interviewed whose music and public persona I had come to dislike and think was bad for the New York hip-hop scene in general, and some underground rappers with whom I was friends had come to share this sentiment, too. The guy was getting played on local radio a lot and seemed to have a lot of industry connections, so it had begun to seem like his ascendance was a foregone conclusion. Given that everyone I knew thought he sucked and that I was also pretty sure that my popping off about him online wouldn't really affect his career (this is one of the keys to being a digital takedown artist—always punch up), one day, on a whim, I dashed off a quick article in which I casually attempted to dismantle his entire existence. I got the idea to write the thing around eleven in the morning; I spent two hours writing it, another hour waiting for a friend to read it so that I could incorporate that feedback, and it was up by three thirty.

Within thirty minutes of pressing "publish," the article had slingshotted out of my orbit and into the galaxy. The local rap station, the one that had been pushing the guy, decided to read the article live on air, and as the story goes, the rapper in question happened to be driving around the city in his car "with the station on" so he drove to the "studio," demanded to be interviewed, and proceeded to say some threatening stuff about me that may have been exacerbated by the on-air personalities asking if he would "retaliate" against me. I was very excited that all of this was happening and found it very funny, and good for sucking more space junk into my orbit. I happened to be DJing at a bar in Brooklyn the following night, so I posted the flyer for the event on Twitter to show exactly how seriously I took the guy. But then he actually took me up on my tacit invitation, and when I took a break from playing music to take in the night air with my friend Gabe, a big guy came up behind me, punched me in the head, yelled "WHAT!" a couple of times in order to make a point, and then jumped into a cab that mysteriously materialized next to him on the street. Three days later, a doctor told me that the man's fist had broken a small bone in my ear and I probably wouldn't be able to hear so well out of it for a few months. On the way back to work, I called a rapper friend and, holding the phone up to my good ear, started telling him about what had happened. But I didn't need to, and we both knew it. The news about the punch had made the rounds on Twitter before bubbling up to random rap blogs and then not-so-random rap blogs, until I, in my most humiliating and painful moment, had become the exact same sort of blip-on-the-radar story that I spent my days writing about. I was spiraling and felt like death. I asked the rapper friend if I was going to die. He laughed and said no. "It's just if you talk enough shit, somebody's gonna smack you." Which, fair enough.

To use the language of addiction, this was probably my "bottom" in terms of being Extremely Online. Like, I didn't *have* to write that article. I just had to write *an* article. Taking the vague feeling around me that this rapper was a hack trying to scam his way into success and rendering that sentiment in the strongest possible terms was my decision, one that the delusion of my online career had convinced me was my civic duty. The company I worked for would make a rounding error's worth more money than it was already going to make because of my writing it, and besides, the people in my little solar system, planets and space junk and moons alike, would all be happy if I wrote it. I never thought about what the other solar systems might make of it. People who say the internet isn't real don't really understand the internet. Instead, the internet is a part of reality, and if you're not careful, you can feel the consequences ringing in your ear.

There's a saying that good entrepreneurs shouldn't be afraid to fail in public, but as someone who failed at not getting punched in the head in public, I can confidently say that this is an objectively insane way to live your life. It's not that failure is inherently shameful; it's just that when we fail in public, there's a greater likelihood that we'll have to explain ourselves rather than simply allow the failure to sit with us. Relearning golf, meanwhile, offered me a *great* opportunity to fail in private.

As I traversed the hills of my local course, alone except for the sounds of nature and the *blump-blump-blump* of my clubs rattling against one another in the bag against my back, I felt jarred by the stillness of it all. In some very real way, I had forgotten what it meant to be truly by myself. For years, I'd pushed off my anxieties by hopping on my phone and tweeting some dumb stuff or pulling up an article that was the literary equivalent of junk food. But on the course, I was able to genuinely engage with my own mind, ask myself why I do the things I do. Eighteen holes is a lot of walking, and there was no one else to have a conversation with to fill the time.

There were times when, between my wobbly grasp on the game and my newfound sense of self-examination, it was too much. Like when I sliced my third ball into the woods while in the middle of a long argument with myself about whether I was a coward for leaving Los Angeles behind for a life of therapy and golf. The rational, accepting, and self-loving part of my brain had finally managed to remind its panicky, anxious other half that admitting I wasn't happy and actually doing something about it was in fact brave, but when I lost that third ball, I felt like a popped balloon. *But it's just golf*, I reminded myself, *and besides, I found that ball in the woods last week*. I laughed at the absurdity of it all, suddenly grounded. No one was judging me about *anything*. It was OK.

• • •

So much of modern life is about living with the illusion that we're free because we have the ability to make choices. But it's the choices themselves that are the mechanisms of control. There are always rules, constraints, character limits, the option to only swipe left or right, react with an emoji of a heart or a little green circle that's vomiting yet still manages to look cute. Technology tells us not what but *how*—how to engage, how to conduct ourselves within an environment, how to pay, how to post. Everything connected to the internet runs on software that communicates via code that is based on a series of ones and zeros: yes or no, up or down, good or bad, following the law or defying it. It's only natural that this either-or mentality would filter up into the way we use these apps and infect our brains.

Online, time seems to dissipate. How many of us have had the experience of mindlessly flicking through our feeds, reading our friends' posts, clicking on articles, chasing down facts on Wikipedia, poking around different sites for a slightly lower price on a pair of sweatpants that we're only half-considering buying? There's no sense of beginning and end to these cycles; they exist only in an ever-elasticizing present. The reason people casually refer to these time-independent jaunts through cyberspace as "K-holes" is that they have the same effect as taking a shitload of ketamine: We dissociate, becoming heads floating on a stick, connected only to a pair of thumbs, passively watching ourselves zip through the internet on autopilot with no idea when the plane is scheduled to land.

Golf, meanwhile, is all about discrete markers of progress. Rounds of eighteen holes divide into front and back nines, which are divided into holes with tee box, fairway, rough, hazards, and green; we measure them in yards, and traverse those yards of these holes with strokes and putts, which we mark on a scorecard. A golf score, then, can be seen as a representation of our journey through time and space—the things that remind us we are present in an environment. On the internet, with its potentially infinite audience, we're never quite sure what will happen to our words and deeds once we put them out there. This can be part of the thrill of being really into posting, but mainly it just makes you go nuts. Conversely, the consequences of every decision on the golf course are plain as day. From the tee box, I might select my driver in the hope that my ball will fly as close to the green as possible, but I increase my risk that I'll slice my shot into oblivion. If the hole is short, or there's a score-killing hazard in play, I might instead tee off with my three-wood or four-iron, which won't go nearly as far but also won't ruin my hole if I hit a terrible shot. But golf is not always a logical game, which is one of the things that make it great. When I'm actually playing, my choices are based off feel more than anything else. I might know that my driver is statistically less accurate than my four-iron, but sometimes you just gotta let it rip and see what happens. And most of the time, knowing that I'm going to hit a good shot somehow creates one, while nerves and pessimism lead to disaster. It runs counter to the nature of probability, or maybe it just speaks to the feebleness and fallibility of the human mind, but it feels like magic, not logic, a reminder of the rewards that come with being comfortable and confident in your body as it exists.

The internet is tricky because it *seems* like a real environment, and it's true that the things we do on the internet have consequences in our daily lives. But the internet has flourished because it's a great way to make money off people, even when they don't realize it. Right now, I'm writing this in Google Docs. It is the website that I spend the most time on, and it has probably been as such for the past decade. Google knows this, and I'm sure that it measures the amount of time I spend actively typing in Docs versus pausing my writing to look for things online via its search engine, and even if it doesn't directly read what I write while using its software, it can probably guess what this book is about merely because of the multiple three-to-five-minute breaks in writing I take to google golf-related things. I give Google my time, attention, and data, all of which, when run through a tech company's algorithms, adds up to money. Even our feelings are worth money to tech companies, because if the internet pushes our buttons in the right ways, we will return to the scene of the crime in an attempt to try to make sense of it all.

I'm not saying that this is bad, necessarily—it may be unavoidable at this point, so there's no sense in moralizing either way—but I want to point out the hidden nature of our relationship with this little yet big non-world that enjoys such purchase over our lives. The golf course puts everything on front street. We know how much it costs to walk onto one. Its rules, however confusing, are made plain to us, and the choices we must make once we're there are obvious, even if there is never really an objectively optimal decision. When I'm out on the course, my focus is entirely on myself. This isn't selfish; rather, it's necessary. We give so much of ourselves away for free online, in the form of our time, energy, emotions, data, words, and all else, that we *need* a place to be private.

We never quite master that which we learn about online—we obtain data and move on, with little regard for how much we may have internalized it. Consider what it would be like to look over the instructions for assembling an IKEA dresser, then hiding them before trying to actually put the thing together. Surely, we would quit out of frustration. The reason the instructions work is that as we follow along with them, we're actually building the thing, forging mental connections between the things on a page and the things in our hands. In real time, we learn what goes where, which techniques we can deploy to secure and stabilize things, or how much pressure to apply to some poor screw before realizing that it's the wrong size and we need to go back a step and figure out what we did with that slightly smaller screw that came in the same little plastic baggie. By the time we're finished, we feel like we're little artisans, our sense of accomplishment making up for the fact that the dresser might be a little uneven and that there are a couple of extra holes where there shouldn't be any. The internet is blind IKEA assembly; golf is learning as we go and being proud that we did the thing at all.

It's rumored that Tiger Woods was taught by his dad, Earl, to hypnotize himself on the golf course so that he could get in "the zone"—whatever mental place allowed him to shoot impressively low scores. This story is pretty clearly not true, because Tiger Woods is not a wizard. Still, there's something to it, if only because playing golf *encourages* a feeling of deep, borderline hypnotic focus that we're often so lacking in the age of smartphones. And until you've been there, it's hard to fully appreciate the contrast between "I must be constantly reachable, constantly aware of what's going on" and "I'm just going to leave my phone on silent until I'm done playing golf." We could always be looking at something more interesting, distressing, or exciting than what's in front of us, but every time we whip our phone out while playing, it breaks the groove that we cultivate from one shot to the next, causing our swings to falter, our hands to shake, our minds to wander when they ought to be governing it all. Experience the havoc wrought by this broken spell enough times, and soon the temptation to check in on the outside world dissipates. In other words, golf encourages one to be fully present.

In her book *How to Do Nothing*, Jenny Odell talks about shrinking her world through immersing herself in birdwatching, writing, "At some point, the impossibility of paying attention to the discrete category [of] 'birds' became apparent. There were simply too many relationships determining what I was seeing." She likens this awakening to learning a new language—in other words, a new set of tools for looking at and navigating the world. Similarly, the golf course is a place where everything—every surface, every object we touch, everything we see and hear and feel—is imbued with meaning, and as golfers, we try to master the cause-and-effect relationships between all of them. So little as shifting our clubface two degrees open at address and slightly dropping the back foot can cause a shot to fly on a right-to-left draw trajectory; even a couple of inches' difference between the level of the ground we're standing on and that upon which the ball rests puts in motion a host of tiny recalibrations of stance, grip upon the club, bend of the knee. This is to say nothing of how our strategy on a hole is shaped by factors such as the height of the grass, the direction and speed of the wind, the slope of the ground, the temperature, the amount of sweat upon our hands.

In this sense, we're a little like Charles Baudelaire's *flâneurs*, those people who walked the streets of Paris and derived otherworldly pleasure from quite worldly observations. The flâneur, he wrote in his essay "The Painter of Modern Life," is a "passionate spectator" with an "eagle eye," a combination of dandy, philosopher, and artist, who views the world through the eyes of a child or a drunk, or both. He compares the flâneur to "a kaleidoscope gifted with consciousness, responding to each one of its movements and reproducing the multiplicity of life and the flickering grace of all elements of life," adding that flâneurs love "to see the world, to be at the center of the world, and yet remain hidden from the world."

When Baudelaire conceived of the flâneur, modern life was exciting. It was the 1860s, and Paris was probably the best place in the world. The city was in the middle of a period of reinvention. Emperor Napoleon III personally funded public works projects meant to turn Paris into *the* cutting-edge city of Europe, with gas lamps illuminating the streets at night and trains coming from everywhere, bringing just about everyone. Paris's population was in the process of doubling in size, and these new people, their thoughts and actions and bodies in constant motion around and against one another, brought new ideas to art and literature and philosophy. Anyone could be anything, and within this revolution of the mind, it was possible to see even the ancient or quotidian with fresh eyes. The flâneur's self-appointed task was to walk the streets of Paris, documenting this sea of humanity, mentally connecting the dots among seemingly disparate people, places, and events, trying to solve the mystery of it all. Clues might range from the curvature of the letters on a hand-painted sign, the expression on a woman's face as she drank a glass of wine alone, the distant sound of a dog's bark, or the sudden destruction of a boardinghouse whose history stretched past the realm of memory. Each of them was related, for the mystery was Paris itself.

For golfers, instead of the city, we have the links. It's this zone between the natural and the artificial, where puddles and deliberate variations in the curvature of the earth take over from the pompous merchant or the wailing toddler. In contrast, the internet is flat, a series of connected nodes that we tap into and navigate. It's rare that we encounter something truly new there; at best, we find sites, videos, images, memes, articles, posts, and the like, which are simply slightly different versions of things we have already seen. If being online feels slightly unfulfilling, then it may very well be because there's only so much room for surprise.

When we golf, meanwhile, we become scholars of landscape without even realizing it, for every shot we hit is shaped by the environment, and it is an environment constructed explicitly for discovery. As we get to know a course, we learn to see the shots we wish to manifest with our mind's eye: a 260-yard drive that ignores the leftward bend of the hole, its unrelentingly straight path climbing as it hugs the left side of the fairway until the ball passes the dogleg and begins its rapid descent, dropping with a couple of bounces until it rolls to the rightmost edge of the short grass, from where we can hit our standard 120-yard approach, whose process has become automatic. Or maybe we face a 180-yard par 3 with a sand trap guarding the front of the green and the pin placed on the back, and ask ourselves whether our four- or five-iron is more up to the task. The five flies higher but shorter, risking exposure to the bunker on a mishit, but the four, if we get all of it, may roll off the green into oblivion. So we run through these potential outcomes in our imagination, settling on a platonic ideal of a five-iron struck true and firm but with a little more elevation than might seem advisable, hoping that it lands on the back lip of the bunker, which, with its downward slope onto the green, will guide our ball directly toward the flag. Even when we fail to turn these dreams to reality, nothing truly bad happens—we just have to hit another shot, which we were going to do even if this one worked out beautifully. There is always another chance, and eventually, we will succeed.

To stand up to a golf ball, feet shoulder width apart, our hands gripping the club with the right force in the right places, knees bent, ass aligned parallel to the heels as we feel our weight within our thighs, is ultimately to ask, "Where shall I explore next?" We may find ourselves exploring the middle of the fairway, or someplace significantly more exciting, like the brush or forest or creek side, from which we are rewarded for a misstruck shot with the opportunity to get creative with our next. These are the parts of the golf course that truly shine. Maybe we have a chance to sneak a peek into someone's yard, stealing a glimpse into their life in the process. Or maybe we find ourselves moving a dead tree branch blocking our swing path, only to find a miniature ecosystem living underneath it. I once lost a ball in some tall rough and found a dead rat where I expected to find my Titleist. The course I was playing on doubled as a nature preserve; the website warns about snakes and foxes afoot. I promptly invented a local rule that I dubbed the "snake threat clause" and gave myself a free drop rather than risk a bite or constriction.

Through wandering, we create and document for our own sake and, in the process, discover something about ourselves. The point of golf is to interpret the world that the course places us in, and to act on those interpretations, not to accomplish something momentous but instead merely to progress, to persevere. An understanding earned only through time, experience, and, most of all, attention can come from something as rudimentary as learning to recognize when we're in a trouble spot—maybe our ball is under a grip of tree branches that threaten the flight of our next shot, or we've got five feet between us and the green and feel the pressure to make up for a missed opportunity, to offer one physical and one psychological example—and, therefore, we should just hit a low-running punch-out to play for position, not distance; or sometimes, a putt off the fringe is safer than a flashy, high-flying flop shot. These moments teach us that we can become masters of our worlds, and we've been able to all along, if only we work to shrink the world rather than expand our efforts.

"Genius," Baudelaire wrote while reflecting on the flâneur, is "childhood recovered at will." On the course, alone and unplugged, we can truly grab hold of who we are, or perhaps once were. As the rate of change in the world and in our lives accelerates at an exponential pace, so does the risk that we become alienated from ourselves, succumbing to the unintentional side effect of trying to keep up with it all. Golf is a corrective to all of this, an opportunity to relearn the world and regain our sense of self through being in a place and devoting our entire attention to it. Call it mindfulness plus a workout, or maybe yoga with way more than a mat. It requires a deep understanding of the body, the relationship and regulation of its parts, the controlled windup of the backswing followed by the joyful abandon of release, and an adventurous spirit from which we derive the will to see things through to the end. These are things so rudimentary that we can barely remember developing an awareness of them, yet golf, with all its strangeness, brings them to the forefront of our experience all over again.

We can recall in painful detail the way that the fourth hole on some anonymous course is a par 4 that seems to stretch out forever, with three cascading tiers of fairway dropping down to a creek bordered by a few feet of unkempt grass on either side, before a two-tiered green shoots up as if it had emerged, fully formed, out of the earth. Such observations, divorced from the golf course itself, don't necessarily hold significance. They matter only in the moment, because of how they shape our thoughts, actions, and movements. Yet in being there, doing the thing, we give them meaning, one that is ours, and ours alone.

Chapter Five

HOW GOLF MADE ME A BETTER SON

"DUDE, TURN AROUND, look at the thing!" The thing was a pixelated image of an alligator with a golf ball in its mouth, accompanied by the words "CAUTION, ALLIGATORS," which had replaced a map of the hole on the LCD screen of our cart. The dude in question was my dad, who was driving directly toward a creek, triggering the alligator warning. The exigent issue was that modern golf carts are equipped with these GPS systems that stop the cart's engine if you drive it too far from the fairway or cart path—which, seeing as we were next to what was allegedly an alligator-infested creek, we definitely were. Things were beeping and it felt like being in a very serious, extremely low-stakes version of war.

"Dad, Dad, Dad!" I yelled. "Reverse! Your ball's gone! I'll give you one of mine. Just don't go near the creek, it's too dangerous!"

He cackled and got out of the cart to fish for his ball with a sand wedge. To be clear, we were in North Carolina, 250 miles from the coast. Alligators do not live there. The farthest inland one has ever come in the state, though, is 210 miles, so absence of evidence isn't evidence of absence. I have seen an alligator on a golf course before, with my dad, at an age when it made an impression. "You're on your own," I said, backing the cart up until it resumed normal functions. I would not have done well in 'Nam.

"But why would they slow your cart down if you were actually near one?" my dad asked. He had a point. "I don't care," I told him, "you follow the signs or else you get in trouble. There's a computer chip in this golf cart, and it's saying we're in danger. It knows." We were both yelling, but it was the fun sort of yelling.

We used to not have conversations like this. The yelling was different, grave. Me because I was a teenager and everything carried an existential importance, even if it was just that they'd installed a speed-tracking system beneath the front seat of the car they'd bought me; and he because they'd just bought me a car even though I'd gotten a speeding ticket six months prior, and he was frustrated that I couldn't see that this was actually pretty reasonable, especially since it wasn't like they were using it to track my location or anything. All he wanted was for me to be safe, and all I wanted was to be allowed to attempt to drive a used Honda CR-V so fast that it looked like the broken lines on the highway started blurring together. I'm gonna go ahead and say I was wrong about that one. But at the time, that didn't stop me from storming off to my bedroom and sulking.

In the intervening years, we have both gained perspective on the speed box issue, along with most things involving the two of us. "You know I'm still gonna kick your butt on this hole, right?" he said. He gave up on telling me not to swear at some point while I was in college, but he doesn't really do it himself. He tried to hit a half shot onto the green with his pitching wedge, pounding his club into the ground at impact in a way that I have never seen a golfer under sixty-four do. “Shit,” he said when the ball went next to nowhere, spitting the word out in the cadence of a parrot that’s still familiarizing itself with human language. I missed my bogey putt; one chip shot later, he missed the putt that would have tied us at six strokes each. We laughed at how poorly we were playing.

It’s the rituals of golf he taught me to love. Unloading our clubs from the trunk of his Chrysler and onto the cart, declaring our first shots off the tee “breakfast balls” and hitting new ones, having hot dogs and Gatorades from the clubhouse at the turn. When he was younger, my dad could hit a driver low and straight until it lost steam and drifted upward before coming to rest, softly, in the fairway. It was my favorite magic trick. He kept his tees in a purple Crown Royal bag in the trunk, next to an identical one with his green-repair tools and ball markers. Back then, I never understood how he told them apart. Now that I know that my dad’s been drunk maybe four times in his life, the mystery inside the memory has changed: How did he get the Crown Royal bags at all? Maybe dads in those days were assigned used Crown Royal bags at the hospital, but the practice has faded with the democratization of the tote bag.

• • •

I grew up in the country, in a place called Polk County. It’s in the southwestern part of the state, where the foothills of the Appalachians intersect with total flatness and create a geothermal anomaly where everything’s a little warmer in the winter and a little cooler in the summer. The air is crisp. Nourishing. Restorative. Semi-edible. It’s one of the reasons F. Scott Fitzgerald moved there in the late thirties as he wallowed in depression, carried on at least one affair, and pumped out writing in a little rented cabin just outside town, some of it so good that it made Ernest Hemingway jealous enough to rent the same cabin after Fitzgerald was done with it. Beyond the fact that F. Scott Fitzgerald was physically there for a while, the rest of this falls somewhere between local legend and well-sourced conjecture, but then again, time does that to all that was once demonstrably true or false.

When biomes bump up against each other, though, the collision yields conflict. Stretches of farmland are naturally demarcated by mounds that jut like stubble from the earth's crust. You can drive past fields for what feels like forever, only to have to yank the emergency brake because suddenly you're in the mountains and about to plow straight off the road into a lake. We've got woods so deep that our old money starts with bootlegging and ends with a landscaping business and an $85,000 pickup. There's new money, or rather money that's new to the place. Teslas tailgate tractors on unnecessarily windy roads, and people who recreationally fund political campaigns maintain summer homes here and refuse to believe that wild boars or coyotes might kill their purebred horses while they're up in New York on business; it must be the people they aren't allowed to call rednecks, the ones who hunt and spit brown into empty Gatorade bottles, doing it for revenge. They filmed *Dirty Dancing* out here, plus *The Last of the Mohicans*. The Navy Seals who killed Osama Bin Laden were armed with tomahawks smithed by the same guy who did the axe and knife that Daniel Day-Lewis is running around with on the poster. He lives out here, too—the knife and axe and tomahawk guy, I mean.

Growing up, I had probably fifteen golf courses within a thirty-minute drive of my parents' house. Some of them had been there since Fitzgerald's days, while others would get built up during boom times and lapse into disrepair or affordability in the not-so-boom times. The one I spent the most time at in high school was called Red Fox. It used to be a housing development with a golf course in the middle, but at some point after my youth, the houses took over. Its website has seemingly been taken over by Chinese pornographers, and the last thing the course's management posted on Facebook, prior to the sale that ended its tenure as an actual golf course, was, "Please continue to support our club through this terrible tragedy. Golf is still open daily." The events leading up to the post are ominous and unknowable, kind of like a David Lynch movie.

Golfing was what one did where I grew up, is what I'm trying to say. My dad golfed before that, though. He started before we lived in Polk County, back before I was born, around the time he kicked off his first career, which was in public education. My dad loved working in schools, helping kids, really being there for them. And sometimes, the middle school outside Charlotte where you taught drama needed a coach for the golf team and you were the only teacher with a pickup truck to put all the kids' golf bags in. Like many a youth coach, the main thing he brought to the table was showing up, caring, balancing their need to have an adult in charge with his need to learn how to actually play golf from the kids on the team. Later on, he became a vice principal at one of the local high schools, and he said it was the best job he ever had. He spent most of his first year on the job trying to clear the bats out of the auditorium, and after all the kids went home, he and another vice principal would set up carpet squares onstage and hit golf balls into the curtain. *Thwack*, *thwack*, *thwack* went the balls, much to the bats' dismay. That guy taught my dad that it didn't matter how far you hit it, only that it went straight.

• • •

My tenure as a junior golfer began shortly after Tiger Woods won the 1997 Masters, when a set of junior golf clubs materialized in my parents' garage. I can't remember if I asked my parents for them (I was about to turn eight, so it's possible) or if my dad had taken it upon himself to buy them for me. In the end, it doesn't matter. Because really, the decision was made by the sheer impact that Tiger Woods had during the final round of the '97 Masters, skinny with a self-assured smile, winning his first major tournament so resoundingly that everyone watching knew that the sport was never going to be the same again.

One of the most profound quotes of the twentieth century is a passage from Antonio Gramsci's *Prison Notebooks*, in which the Italian revolutionary wrote, "The old is dying but the new cannot be born; in this interregnum a great variety of morbid symptoms appear." It's pretty famous as far as quotes by dead Italian Communists go, and it's been used to describe everything from America's lagging role in world affairs to public health crises to why Britain shouldn't change its public school system. My interpretation of what Gramsci originally meant is this: Sometimes, change is impossible because even if it's high time for change, if there's dead weight at the top, it ain't gonna happen. And as the energies of change seek their release, the pressure within the system builds up, causing dark and strange things to leak out, each a scream demanding recognition.

By the mid-nineties, professional golfers were in the middle class of professional athletes, if you could even call them that. Pros smoked cigarettes during their rounds, and so many of them played hung over that there was a special putting technique, the "whiskey finger," meant to stabilize their shaky hands on the green. If they won a tournament, they might pocket a quarter of a million dollars or so, rather than the cool million they win on today's tour. The last time a transcendent golfer had touched down on the links was in the early sixties when Jack Nicklaus turned pro, and he was now kicking around the Senior PGA Tour. The old world of golf was dying.

Yet the new wanted to be born. This was also around the time when woods stopped being made out of actual wood, which doesn't sound like that big a deal, but in truth it revolutionized the game. Wooden woods had to be compact, because wood is heavy as hell, which meant that precision took precedence over power off the tee. But once golf companies developed the technology allowing them to create hollow-bodied metal woods, they got bigger and bigger, effectively expanding the sweet spot on the clubface and allowing golfers to swing at the ball with abandon. Golf courses were getting built up like crazy, too, thanks to the economic boom of the Clinton years, and cable companies had just added the Golf Channel to their basic packages. There were means, motive, and opportunity for golf to be reborn.

And in 1997, Tiger Woods pulled the trigger. It wasn't just that he was talented and handsome, or that as a young multiracial man he looked nothing like the old white men he was competing against, although I'd be lying if I said that didn't have something to do with it. Simply by existing, he directly repudiated the sport's long-standing stereotypes, his popularity sometimes forcing the sport to rethink itself in terms of accessibility and equality—which, on occasion, provided the golf establishment with the opportunity to cite him as proof that its issues with accessibility and equality were no longer problems, without actually doing anything to actively correct those issues or atone for the hardships they'd caused in the past. (Woods asked for none of this, and at twenty-one he seemingly wanted to have nothing to do with it, famously going on *Oprah* and rejecting the term "African American" and instead self-identifying as a "Cablinasian.")

Yet for all the pressure placed upon him to single-handedly change the image of golf, Woods won, over and over again, and won in ways that changed how the game was actually played. When he hit the ball, it went and went, and courses got longer in futile attempts to stymie him. Some of this was because of the shift in technology, but beyond that, Tiger was one of the first pro golfers to realize that being an athlete—as in, someone in world-class physical shape—could provide him with an edge.

Beyond that, there was the touch and finesse and pure creativity he brought to the game. Tiger could hit a ball and make it spin sideways when it landed. He had a sixth sense for where to land a chip shot on the green so that it would trickle into the hole, turning bogey to birdie in the process. He once hit a sixty-foot putt dead left of the cup, having calculated the exact point on the green where it would hit a slope and veer right, arcing slowly toward the target until it fell in. It takes a dizzying grasp of the game's physics, combined with an ability to enact those physics at will upon a golf ball, to make all these things happen, but when I watched as a kid, it just seemed like Tiger was steering the golf ball with his brain. And he did it all with a sense of joy. I'll never forget a commercial he cut for Nike, in which he effortlessly bobbles a golf ball off his lob wedge for nearly half a minute. Left hand: bounce, bounce, bounce. Right hand: bounce, bounce, bounce. Between the legs: bounce, bounce, bounce. Behind the back: bounce, bounce, bounce. Catch the ball with the sheer surface of the wedge, displaying a softness of the hands that you cannot teach, then pop it up again to bounce, bounce, bounce. Another bounce, this one high. Tiger takes a full swing and sends the ball sailing away.

• • •

My tenure as a budding junior golfer ended for reasons that have nothing to do with Tiger Woods. I was at a golf camp, not one of the sleepaway ones, because I was scared of those. Every day, we hit balls on the range and learned how to putt and chip. I wasn't good, but I was eight, so that wasn't really the point. It was my first time playing golf around someone who wasn't my dad, and I didn't know any of the kids. One of the pros there would make us do push-ups if we messed up in a drill. He called me Amos like he thought it was my name, but when I grew up, I realized it was because my dad's name is Andy and that was a radio show. This is the purpose of day camps, I think: getting conditioned to creating relationships that fall away after a set period of time. Consider it training for becoming an adult.

But at this golf day camp, I loved more than anything to swing my golf clubs. Big swings. The process of the windup fascinated me on a physical level; I had been a terrible T-ball player because I insisted on doing the full pitcher's windup whenever I fielded a hit and attempted to throw it to the relevant baseman, which started happening a lot because the other coaches picked up on it and told their kids to aim for me. So I did the windup golf swing even when I wasn't supposed to, which caught me some flak from the guy who called me Amos because if I wasn't careful and someone was standing near me or in the path of any golf ball I hit, I could hurt somebody.

One day, when a bunch of kids and I were messing around on the practice green, I did.

Not with an actual golf club. That would have been terrible. In high school, I once saw a kid get hit in the face with a four-iron because of a freak accident, and it was a whole thing involving listening to the sound of cheekbones crunch like a bag of ice cubes as we walked him to the clubhouse so he could go to the hospital and get surgery. I don't think I could have done that to a kid, necessarily, because I was eight and skinny and couldn't swing a club very fast. Maybe I could have given somebody a firm bonk that yielded an alarming bump, preferably not on the head. But I wouldn't have broken anyone's anything.

What I did do was this: My ball was at the bottom of a little green hill. In order to putt it to the cup, I would need to putt it hard. So I putted the ball as if I were trying to drive it into the fairway, which sent the ball screaming off the hill and directly into another kid's ankle. I remember him writhing on the green, crying, and me saying that I was sorry over and over again, meaning it so much that I cried, too. The man who called me Amos told me I needed to sit by myself until my parents got there, as I offered to do as many push-ups as I needed to so he knew how much I wanted to take back what I just did, but he was shaking his head and telling me that sometimes we do things we can't fix by doing push-ups. I was allowed to come back to golf camp the next day, but instead I spent the rest of the week at my grandparents'.

Maybe this was all Tiger Woods's fault. I mean, it was mostly just an unfortunate accident that I brought into being, but Tiger influenced me and millions of other kids to pick up a golf club.

• • •

Fast-forward four years to the summer before I entered seventh grade. The wounds from the incident at golf camp had healed (my mental ones, at least, though I hope the kid's physical ones had as well), and my parents had started letting me watch R-rated movies. The first one was *The Matrix*, because it was ubiquitous and as a middle school boy in the summers before 9/11, if you went to a sleepover, you *would* watch *The Matrix* because it was and continues to be totally badass. After the dam broke, my parents let me watch R-rated movies before the advent of the PG-13 rating. It gave them some sort of plausible deniability from a being-a-good-parent standpoint.

I watched the classics. *National Lampoon's Animal House*. *The Jerk*. *Stripes*. *The Blues Brothers*. *National Lampoon's Vacation*. Eventually, I got to *Caddyshack* and wore out the DVD. I could not join a fraternity or the army. I did not have a brother to form a blues band with. We already had a dog, and my parents wouldn't let me change his name to Shithead. But I had once played golf, and I could, hypothetically, play golf again.

Red Fox was still a golf course back then, and I asked my dad to take me there. The next thing I knew, he was in the basement throwing together a set of clubs for me, loading them into his old golf bag, which was chunky and grass green and had a 7 Up logo on it. When I was a kid, I'd always thought that 7 Up had made golf stuff along with soda because of that bag. Now I knew that this bag was special, and that there were no others like it in the world holding cobweb-covered clubs with the name "Golfsmith" stamped on them. OK, maybe some. But not many.

Into the Chrysler and out to the course, stopping inside the pro shop, a drywall-and-plywood afterthought of a building, to check in. The first hole was a par 5 where you were supposed to hit your tee shot straight into the fairway, then make a ninety-degree right turn to take your second shot over a creek and onto another fairway, and approach with a short iron into the green. First holes are meant to be friendly, and this was doubly so. When I was in high school, we all tried to cut the dogleg by aiming diagonally off the tee and sneaking it over the creek. It worked frequently enough that we kept trying, no matter how many times we didn't hit it far enough and plopped it in the water. But on this, my inaugural round of golf, I did it by accident, slicing the hell out of my drive, the ball landing softly in the rough with a clear shot to the green. One semi-whiff, an unintentionally low-running worm burner, and a gentle chip later, and I was putting for par, then bogey, then sinking my third putt for a double bogey. It was a mess—and I loved it. The possibilities that presented themselves locked their hooks into me until I left for college.

On Saturdays, I played soccer. I was better at it than I was at golf but had less room for improvement. I was slow and skinny and not particularly imaginative when it came to what to do when the ball came my way, but none of these things were issues on the golf course, where I had time to think about my technique and get the shot right. There was a place in the country out near the soccer complex that was a golf shop with a driving range attached, and we'd stop there after games so I could practice hitting balls. It became a routine, to the point where my dad decided to go whole hog and buy me a set of used clubs, old King Cobra Oversize irons plus a couple of Adams Tight Lies fairway woods (the driver came later), as well as some lessons from a pro out in the next town over. He'd have me hit a few shots with my seven-iron while taping it, and then we'd go into his office and play it back to me by running his VCR through a computer, which had a program that allowed him to draw triangles and lines over my body to illustrate the principles of the golf swing, where my body needed to be versus where it was. Back to the range to practice, more video, repeat. Through this, golf became a trigonometric exercise, and whenever puberty wasn't making my body to metamorphose so quickly that I lost all spatial awareness of my limbs, I started playing pretty OK.

Unfortunately, puberty was usually making my body do insane things. My brain, too. The summer between my first and second year of high school, I grew about six inches and couldn't handle it at all. When I walked over the threshold of a door, I would trip on it and fully fall probably half the time. I was frustrated and felt every feeling at once and knew that no one would ever understand how I felt even if I didn't have any particular reason for feeling it. I never knew what to say to people, especially girls, and I got good grades, which somehow made it all worse. Dad and I kept going to Red Fox, probably once a month, and the trips became excruciating.

When I kept a hold over my balance, I would hit the ball great. I could make my seven-iron go where I wanted, and through trial and error on the range, I learned how to sharply draw the ball low and left around corners or out of the woods, which helped me make up for the fact that I couldn't drive the ball to save my life and lacked the patience to learn how to putt well. Sadly, these were the main things that made high school golfers look cool to one another, so I was constantly trying to kill it off the tee, rather than just hitting a nice smooth four-iron to the middle of the fairway, and turning potential bogeys into triples by overpowering every putt farther than five feet. But when I was with my friends, I could take mulligans and concede putts to myself, so I never got better.

Playing with my dad was a different story. "You've got to see it through," he'd say after I'd hit my tee shot into the side of a hill. "It's only your third shot now; it's fine."

In the face of this highly reasonable and valuable patriarchal wisdom, I would, almost inevitably, explode. I'd start saying things in all caps, like "THIS SUCKS I'M QUITTING GOLF FOREVER" and "FUUUUCK" (that one always followed by a decidedly lowercase "oh god dad i'm sorry for cussing"). I was never successful at following through on my intention to quit golf forever, though, because I was in the middle of a golf course and the only thing worse than sucking at golf would be watching my dad golf while I stayed in the cart, stewing in a pre-smartphone ennui that I wonder if teens ever experience anymore.

• • •

There's a process that parents and children go through, in which each party discovers who the other really is. Kids want to please their parents, or at least do things that are in direct conversation with their parents' hopes/wishes/dreams, etc. Parents, meanwhile, have so much love and care and fear and hope and pride and anxiety when it comes to their kids. They are parents, and they want to be good at it, but no one tells them what that actually means (also, it tends to involve deep terror over the physical safety of their kids, which lasts for at least two decades). Parents love their children no matter what, and everything they say and do flows from that, and all that love and fear manifests in a deep desire to be understood by those they love more than anything else. That's what my friends who have kids tell me, at least, and that's what my dad, who at this point is also my friend, and who has a kid, who is me, says, too.

Communication, under the best of circumstances, is hard. Histories pile up, build walls. Create pain points. Cause some things to be all you want to talk about, and cover other stuff up. But on the golf course, with no phones or distractions, the conversation naturally ebbing and flowing thanks to talk of things like club selection and speculation about the slope of the green, those same blocks have a funny way of shaking loose. I've learned to see my father as his own person, who experiences hurt and pain just as I do, and that I myself had caused him hurt and pain in my life, yet he has always loved me unconditionally.

It took years for me to understand that following the hole through to the end, no matter how badly it turns out, to not lose one's cool, to play every shot honestly, giving it all one's focus, isn't just a golf thing. There are things in life that will suck. That do suck.

The older you get, the more of them you will experience. You will learn heartbreak and rejection and what it feels like to not feel good enough, as well as the dangers of feeling way too good. You will be driving across a highway when another car, going too fast and manned by a driver paying too much attention to a phone, will slam into your left rear wheel, sending you spinning all the way to some yard three lanes away. You will work for no money in the most expensive city in America, only to discover you are broke once you learn that the limit on your credit card does not reset every month. You will get picked up by the cops, drunk and shirtless, smoking a cigarette outside your apartment, and it will take you two more years to realize that this is a sign that you still have some growing up to do. You will be bitten in the face by a pit bull and receive stitches in the apartment of an off-duty ER doctor. You will sign up for a rafting trip with your partner, only to have an anxiety attack during the onshore safety talk because you're a terrible swimmer, be told by the guide that it's too late to bail, and subsequently fall out of the boat and slide under the surface, losing control in the rapids, scraping your knees and shins and hands on the slick, sharp crags beneath you as you gasp and flail, but discover that after a lifetime of fear you can, in fact, open your eyes underwater, and this allows you to see a big rock coming up on your side that you can wedge both your hand and foot into, allowing the rescue crew—there is a rescue crew by now—to catch up and fish you out.

Your father knows that these things will happen, not because he is clairvoyant but because he has lived his own version of them, and while the details may differ, the pain is always the same. He wants to protect you from having to go through it all, but he knows he can't, because the older you get, the more these things just happen as a matter of course. So he teaches you to take your penalty strokes, because life is often arbitrary and tragic, and there are no mulligans when things don't work out. You hit the ball. It goes the wrong way again, but it's playable, and after hitting your shots into the woods and then out and then onto the green (finally), you end up with a quadruple bogey. You are enraged, but when you get older, you'll understand.

Chapter Six

HOW GOLF MADE ME A BETTER FRIEND

OVER THE YEARS, I've developed a theory that without proper care and feeding, our social lives trend toward entropy. You make friends in high school, and if you all stay in town or go away for a while and then move back, great. But usually, they move or you move or both. Same thing with college, only more so: By the time you graduate, you've amassed a Rolodex of friends, acquaintances, roommates, classmates, enemies, townies, crushes, exes—this entire vibrant social world. And it stays with you, at least parts of it do, as you graduate and go out into the world and work, find your niche, join a scene, and generally try to navigate your twenties and thirties. Between your college friends and your new ones, your social world compresses, little by little, as you get older and responsibilities pile up and your actual world expands, this time full of strangers, while the bonds of your past shrivel until only a small core remains.

Then one day, you drive past a friend's house and knock on the door, just to say *Hi*. They must be home. They're always home.

But then no one answers, so you call them, and they're buying art supplies. They're an artist? They've made art for money for the past two years. You'd have known that if you'd stopped by more often. But they hadn't stopped by, either. Because they were making art, following their passion while you followed yours. These things happen and they're nobody's fault, but you start noticing them more and more. And sometimes when you reconnect, it's better and deeper, but far far far too often, it's just not the same. Whatever commonality you once shared is gone now, and the best you can hope for is a nostalgic walk down memory lane, waving to the person you used to be.

You've been reading this book long enough to know what I'm going to propose as a solution to this issue, so I won't say the thing you know I'm going to say just yet. Instead, I'll point out that relationships, no matter the type, are forged around something—conversations, activities, histories, common bonds both social and otherwise. The reason it's easy to make friends in college is that you see everyone all the time, and the law of averages says if you're around enough people for a long enough time, you're bound to find yours. In a new city, in a new job, with a new schedule, that all melts away. Social mores change. People become suspicious of one another. If you see people at a bar wearing the T-shirt of a band you like, you can't just go up and talk to them. It's weird, and besides, they're with their friends and you're with yours, and none of you have the desire to slide out of your comfort zone and into the unknown.

This is probably technology's fault, too. Smartphones and the internet have lowered the opportunity costs of keeping in touch down to just a few seconds and some taps, or at least that's how it feels when we're the ones doing the tapping. But the difference between sending someone a compliment in the form of a liked post and offering a thoughtfully specific, sincerely delivered positive comment is everything. One is a product of its medium, while the other cannot be fully communicated electronically. And how many times have you gone up to an acquaintance at a party and felt at a loss for words because you know the person just went on vacation, or got engaged, or started a new job, because of something that was posted? Asking how someone has been, or what the acquaintance has been up to, feels more artificial than usual, but straight-up asking, "Hey, how was Barbados?" implies an unearned familiarity the likes of which has made us cringe when we've been on the receiving end of it. And so instead, you drink your drink, make eye contact, exchange nods, and turn around in an attempt to find someone you're already close with or don't know at all, anything but anyone who's in between.

Those dating apps where you swipe left or right on people's photos are an example of this in microcosm. The stated point of the apps, obviously, is to help people meet partners—long-term, casual, and everything in between. But if you actually *do* find a person you're happy with, then you cease to use the apps yourself, which—even though a few pitch themselves as "the dating app to be deleted" or something like that—is doubly obviously bad for their business. Often, what happens is a person matches with someone, the two go on a date that feels forced and awkward because of the innate pressure of meeting a stranger, compounded with a complete lack of common bonds, and then, dejected, they both get back on the apps and start swiping as soon as they get home. I've known people who've become almost addicted to this pattern, using the apps to set up multiple dates a week, sometimes multiple dates in a single evening, becoming so focused on the act of setting up and going on dates that they can't possibly get to know anyone. It's human nature to fail to focus on what's in front of us when we know something else is out there.

The internet passes itself off as a cure for loneliness, but it does so by masking the fact that often the internet itself is actually causing that same loneliness. No one designed its individual parts to function that way when put together, but it's an ecosystem whose push-pull adds to its habit-forming tendencies. We have so many new ways to make plans, but it gives us even more reasons to break them, from last-minute work emails to breaking news that's never not horrifying, to simply a nagging sense that by ungluing ourselves from our screens, we might miss out on something worth seeing, or knowing, or bearing witness to in real time. All of this adds to a sensation that when we're plugged in, we're participating, but most of the time, the two-way street is only an illusion. We comment and post, but are told, implicitly and explicitly, about what to say and how. Besides, other people can be a bust. But there's always something crazy going down online.

OK, here's the thing you know I was going to say: Golf is like a hot razor cutting through the butter of acquaintanceship straight to the heart of true friendship. I think about this a lot because of Troy, a person I had known for years through mutual friends, with whom I'd often casually chatted about nonsense in bars and backyards. One evening, this time in the backyard of a bar (oh, the variety offered to people in their early thirties!), I offhandedly mentioned my golf addiction to Troy's fiancée, only for her to holler to him from a couple of tables over. He, too, was under the game's thrall, and from there, it was off to the races. Eyes lit up. Numbers were exchanged. Plans were discussed, first in the abstract, then drilling down into the specifics. We'd made the jump from semi-friendship to the realm of the real.

While golfing alone has its charms, allowing us access to our unfiltered interiority, it's also very much a social game. On the course with others, you've got to fill the silence somehow, whether it's by going deep with each other or simply shooting the breeze. After a few rounds together, usually brain-breakingly early weekend outings, I learned that Troy and I had a lot in common. We both loved old Memphis hip-hop, watched the same shows, and were inconsistent golfers, capable of joyous highs on the course that erased our numerous lows. He had stories about convincing his biology-professor neighbor to retrieve a snake from his garden, about the day he accepted that he was going bald and taught himself how to shave his head, about making his only hole in one thanks to a bad shot that ricocheted off a bunch of rocks, only to land on the green and roll into the hole.

We liked golfing together, and we wanted a regular excuse to do it. So we decided to form a golf team and join a league. Troy conscripted his work friend Whitaker onto the team, while I got my buddy Luke, who probably technically qualified as a ringer in that he was a certified PGA professional, on board. Luke wasn't an actual pro or anything, just a guy who worked in the golf industry. You have to take a test, and it's hard, but it's way different from being a person who makes money playing tournaments.

But I digress. The golf league became a perfect excuse for all of us to get together: nine holes, once a week, for nine weeks, and with only two of our scores counting each hole, the ideal amount of pressure (aka zero) to boot.

You learn a lot about people while playing golf with them. Do they check their stance before they swing? Do they use their practice swing to test how their ball's lie will affect the shot? How far can they hit the ball versus how far do they *think* they can hit the ball? What happens when they hit a good shot? A bad one? Do they keep things simple and safe, or do they try to get all fancy and take a high-risk shot that requires expert technique? Do they care about putting, or do they view it as a minor annoyance standing in the way of the very fun business of hitting the ball far? (For the record, I often forget to check my stance, am more focused on taking only one practice swing than on taking a practice swing that would actually help me, think that I hit my shots shorter distances than I actually do, am gracious when complimented on good shots, laugh at bad shots, and fastidiously practice my putting on a mat at home.)

Through playing together, I discovered that both Troy and I are apologizers. Despite always trying to maintain good cheer even when I'm playing bad golf, a few double bogeys in a row breaks the dam and sends the sorries gushing out. Meanwhile, Troy let his own ones out reflexively, getting so much into the habit of apologizing when he'd miss a putt that it'd bleed into his repertoire whenever we'd just play together for fun. What was funny is that nobody on our team was judging anyone else for screwing up—whoever won our league got a free round of golf at our home course, which cost all of thirty bucks, plus entry into a tournament whose prize was going to be a poster designed by Luke's company. We were just there to have fun. Troy reminded me of this whenever I said sorry for slicing, and I'd do the same for him, but nonetheless, apologize we did.

Whitaker and Luke, the two strongest players on the team, each developed his own strategy for success. Luke began the season playing with hundred-year-old, hickory-shafted golf clubs, each much more difficult to hit with than any club that's been made since the Cold War. There's an entire scene out there full of hickory enthusiasts who get together for tournaments, give each other advice on refurbishing ancient thrift-store finds, keep up with each other on forums. Some seem to think that it's the purest way to play the game, while others just think it's cool and weird and therefore good. Once, while I was playing with Luke, the face of his ancient seven-iron (or, to use the preferred term, mashie niblick) got caught up in a bit of soggy fairway and caused the wooden shaft to snap in half. But a month later, I'd learn, those same hickory-shafted clubs, repaired mashie niblick included, got run over by a pickup truck along with a few newer clubs he had. Only the hickories survived.

Luke once described himself to me as a "golf club hoarder," and for him, part of the fun was testing out toys, whether old or new. Each week of the season, a different club would find its way into his bag. First, there was a gigantic driver that he'd use to pop the ball unfathomably far, then a couple of shiny wedges for around the green, a hybrid that seemed to be every single shade of neon, and finally, a set of irons, spit-shined save for the rusted-out spots in the centers of their faces.

As the season wore on, he became the devil on my shoulder, on nearly every tee box getting a wild look in his eyes and whispering, conspiratorially, "Hit driver." While I'm much more accurate with a three-wood or a hybrid, the driver is *way* more fun, even if (or maybe because?) using it puts me at risk of ruining my entire round. Luke wanted to see highlights from his teammates. It's fun to play with someone like that, whose view of the game is divorced from numbers and instead looks at golf more like, I don't know, skiing, in which adrenalizing success erases all failure.

Whitaker, meanwhile, quickly earned the nickname "Mr. Consistent" by always staying out of trouble and never failing to send his shots straight. He was automatic: Plop the ball out in the fairway, plop the ball onto the green, plop it toward the hole, then plop it in; wash, rinse, repeat. He rarely scored worse than bogey, and his lack of pyrotechnics made it easy to forget how good he truly was—that is, until we'd check the scorecard at the end of the round. His job became locking in pars so that Troy, Luke, and I could try dumb nonsense that might notch us a birdie—think attempting to drive the green on par 4s, gunning for chip-ins that could very easily leave us off the green if we didn't sink them, trying to bend balls around trees toward the green instead of simply punching out—stuff that, if and when we screwed it up, often left us facing down triple bogeys. But with Whit there, only one of us actually had to pull it off.

My favorite teammate to watch play, though, was Troy, who treated golf with arch nonchalance. While the rest of us indulged in complex practice swing routines and, while addressing the ball, attempted to hone our minds to focus upon the task at hand, Troy simply stepped up, took his club halfway back to engage his muscle memory, and let it rip. He never minded us talking during his swing; hell, he may have even played better while talking during his *own* swing. To Troy, it was all about the unconscious nature of the game, letting feel take the wheel and staying so out of the moment that he was able to make an end run around his ego and hum along with the unconscious. One day, on a par 5, he hooked his drive into the woods, snaked his ball out and through the fairway into the opposite rough, pitched it over the green, and chipped back to within six inches of the hole to save par.

As the season wore on, we learned that our styles complemented one another's perfectly. Whitaker kept the train running, Luke served as the power hitter, Troy became the miracle worker, and I ended up being the utility player, adapting my game to fit the situation at hand. Sometimes I pulled out my driver and let loose, sometimes I tried to keep it in the fairway and make at worst a bogey, sometimes I did trick shot stuff, and when left to my own devices, I tried to keep my score down however I could. Each week, our team's scores improved. It wasn't that any of us got dramatically better, but instead that we learned how to support one another within the context of the two-best-scores-per-hole format, working to manage risk and reward on each hole and encouraging one another to favor our strengths whenever it was our individual time to shine. Whitaker always teed off first, then Troy and Luke, then me: If the middle two dudes hit one of their shots to the short grass, then I was free to go deep; if not, I grabbed my three-wood and opted for the safe play. When one of us had messed up and wouldn't be getting anywhere near par, we'd try to position our ball on the green near that of the person who had the best chance of scoring low so that they could learn from the way our putt rolled and have a better chance of sinking their own. In other words: We discovered ways to turn the ultra-individualistic game of golf into a genuine team sport.

And that's how, in the penultimate week of the competition, we found ourselves in first place, seemingly cruising to victory. The afternoon of our round, Luke got stuck in traffic and showed up maybe a minute before we were supposed to start; another team helped themselves to our tee time without asking. In the abstract, this wasn't necessarily that big a deal: There were four of them, there were four of us, so it seemed like we'd each play at the same pace. Except that those guys, a squad of middle-aged hackers, sucked. A lot. On nearly every hole, they'd get stuck in the sand and spend multiple shots trying to pitch out, accidentally putt off the green, or hit it out of bounds and have to take a two-stroke penalty and try again. OK, no judgment. I'd done all that stuff before, and definitely did it while playing in that league. Golf is hard, and stakes, even very low ones, can make it even harder.

This is where the mental element of the game comes in. Part of the fun is overcoming the pang of anguish that accompanies a bad shot and finishing out the hole. That was the entire point of how we played, but we soon found out that not everyone agreed with us—namely, the slow-playing villains who'd skipped past us in line. As we watched them pile up strokes on every hole, we killed time by checking the league's app where each team publicly posted its score, only to discover —

"Hey, wait a second," Whitaker said, passing his phone around.

"What the hell?" I said when it came my way. Despite what was happening right before our eyes, according to the scoreboard app, the team in front of us was playing fantastically, posting pars and birdies like nobody's business. By the seventh hole, our team was collectively three strokes over par—while these guys were at even par.

We dug into the app some more. Their scores for the day's round were a statistical anomaly when compared with their prior rounds, but the way that the league's points system worked, there existed a scenario in which they could win both this week—which they were well on the way to doing—and the following week's final round, racking up enough points in two weeks to potentially win the league championship. We calculated that even though we were currently leading the league, if we came in second today and third the week after, we would lose to our new rivals—and we became so focused on teasing out every possible scenario that we ended up getting a collective double bogey on a par 3.

Their sudden breakthrough seemed fishy. Luke snuck off to spy on them, which wasn't very sportsmanlike. However, desperate times call for pulling some shady maneuvers, even if you're the person who's furnishing the prize that lies at the end of the road. Through a little thicket of trees separating the seventh fairway from the eighth, Luke counted their strokes. Six, five, seven, five. They marked down a pair of fours.

The Monday before the final round, our team group chat ignited. *I made a spreadsheet lol*, Whitaker texted, attaching a screenshot of a neatly arranged Excel document containing our rivals' scores on each hole for each round of the season, strategically bolding last week's data to indicate its status as a statistical aberration. He emailed the data he'd compiled to the league coordinator, along with a complaint about the other team's unsportsmanlike conduct. While this could arguably be classified as "snitching" and therefore very lame, we were snitching on four affluent dads, so by my estimation, it's actually class warfare or intergenerational conflict. The point is, the league admin guy saw all this stuff and was like, *Oh yeah that does look weird, I'll tell them to knock it off*, and that was that.

This is all stupid and kind of petty, but there are worse fires in which to forge the bonds of friendship. We didn't *really* care, but our shared and very silly struggle gave us an opportunity to bond. We ended up winning the final round, handily and anticlimactically so. The other team, suitably chastened, didn't cheat this time, and we ended up playing as well as we had all season. We did the thing, and things were good.

• • •

In the weeks following our victory, tragedy of the utterly quotidian variety struck.

The fancy-schmancy golf course attached to UNC–Chapel Hill, which was set to host the tournament that we'd get to play in for winning our league title, announced that it was broken. As in: Over spring, summer, and fall, the place had been packed to the gills with golfers dropping $80 a pop to play there, creating so much traffic that the course itself languished. The greens became fuzzy and unmown, the traps left unraked and accumulating rocks. Fairway divots from the previous March, never filled in, grew over, leaving each hole speckled with inch-deep depressions in the earth that only a masochist would hit out of.

Someone once told me that playing a great golf course is like savoring a fine wine. If so, then UNC's had devolved into a box of Franzia that had been drained to the point where nothing comes out when you tap it except for a sad sucking sound. So the course was closed for maintenance. It was supposed to be for only two weeks, just enough time to cut the things that needed cutting and regrow the things that needed regrowing, hypothetically yielding a rejuvenated golf course opening on the day of the tournament. But you can't dictate the schedule on which a golf course heals, because you're simply a facilitator. Constructions of humanity though they are, golf courses are living things, biomes that ebb and flow at their own pace.

All of which is to say that come tournament time, the course still wasn't open and the organizers, in their infinite wisdom, postponed the thing.

But Troy, Whit, and I had already taken off work that day, so instead we decided to all play together somewhere else. I googled "best golf courses in NC" and went down some website's list, calling the close-ish ones to see if they had any tee times available. Forty-two courses down the page, I successfully booked us a round of golf. The forty-second-best course in the state is nothing to sneeze at, and it turned out to be the perfect combination of nice, challenging, laid-back, and "sells beer."

In between holes, we talked about houses because my partner, Emilie, and I were about to buy one. "You're going to hate whoever owned your house last," Troy said. "Because everyone's so weird and they do shit to a place that no one else would possibly think to do." In his case, the previous owner installed the heating system himself and had no idea what he was doing; they bought in the summer and discovered in the winter that everything was loose and mis-wired and a pretty definite fire hazard. I told them about how my aunt and uncle once got a place where the knobs on some bedroom doors were reversed so the locks were on the outside, presumably because the previous owners had poorly behaved kids whom they'd decided to (more or less) jail. "Every room in our new spot is painted an insane color," Whitaker said. "Every weekend, we pick a room and paint it. It's fun to have something to do together."

• • •

When I'm old and decrepit, my adult grandchildren looking at me, unable to think of anything but the inevitable day they'll have to upload what's left of my mind to the Cloud, they will attempt to stave off these terrible visions by asking me what it was like to be young when I was young. With what little strength I still have left, I will smile, and I will tell them about Four Loko.

In college, you party because you are, for perhaps the first time in your life, truly alive. You are no longer ruled by your parents, so you party because those totalitarian old people raised you to act responsibly, and partying is not responsible. You have no experience, but partying will give you experience of a sort, memories that will feel meaningful and transgressive in their immediate aftermath, but that will in time come to seem risky and regrettable. To party is to slip into a second skin, belonging to someone who is witty and dynamic, confident, fearless, incapable of making a bad decision. You ignore those who say you are a mumbling, reckless idiot, because you are a superhero and they are just jealous they can't keep up whenever you take to the skies. You are beholden to nothing and no one—not even, if you party hard enough, yourself. This impulse—to let loose, to get out of your own head, to willfully enact chemical imbalances in pursuit of transcendence—has been present in humanity since time immemorial, and it will remain long after we are all dead.

But for a brief and shining moment in the mid- to late 2000s, this impulse had a name, and that name was Four Loko. For $3, you were not simply buying a highly alcoholic, moderately caffeinated beverage that tasted like stomped-up Jolly Ranchers mixed with Drano—you were effectively purchasing a license to act insane.

When my dad was a kid, he saw an ad for some PF Flyers athletic shoes, which boasted that the wearer would be able to run faster and jump higher. He saved up his allowance for weeks, all in the service of buying the sneakers that would let him perform at a new level. And what happened the day he finally bought them and decided to test them out by leapfrogging over the glass table in his parents' living room? He crashed right through it and had to get a bunch of stitches.

At its peak, Four Loko was the alcoholic beverage equivalent of PF Flyers. That is, if the shoes had actually worked. Again, we're talking about a drink that cost $3 and had a word that translated to *crazy* in its name. (Or perhaps the name was a winking reference to Loki, the Norse trickster god who, according to the estimable Norse-Mythology.org, once resolved a problem by tying "one end of a rope to the beard of a goat and the other end to his testicles," which is an extremely Four Loko thing to do.) If it wasn't for the fact that it gave you a hangover *while* you were drinking it, the drink would have been perfect.

Four Loko stories tend to come in a few flavors: Loko-induced property damage, Loko-induced public indecency, Loko-induced hospitalizations, and Loko-induced friendly wrestling that quickly devolved into all-out brawling. Four Loko once told the brain of a friend of mine to tell his body to jump onto the hood of a Mercedes and smash its windshield with a skateboard. Somebody once told me they knew a guy who drank a couple of Lokos at a basement punk show and moshed so hard that he accidentally made the house cave in.

As anecdotes like these, both real and exaggerated, piled up on social media and in the press, Four Loko in its caffeinated form became a public health concern, to the point that New York Senator Chuck Schumer called for it to be banned in his home state. Under increasing pressure, the drink's maker, Phusion Projects, announced it would be decaffeinating its signature product in November 2010. But we all get the caffeine taken out of us at some point. We grow old and we lose the wildness within us and there is nothing we can do about it, but that is a good thing because the wildness is what can hurt us and others around us. We regain control of our impulses, channel them in healthy directions. Again, you probably know the direction I'm talking about here. But for now, pretend that you don't.

The story of the dumbest thing I ever did in college started when my friend handed me several hundred dollars in cash and asked me to drive to the nearest convenience store to buy the place out of Four Loko. It was fall 2010, and college campuses were abuzz with rumors that the government was going to ban the sale of energy drinks that contained alcohol, or maybe alcoholic beverages that contained caffeine—we weren't really all that sure. But no matter the specifics, it seemed imperative that my friend—we'll call him Steve—ask me to buy so much still-caffeinated Four Loko that it made the trunk of my Volvo scrape the curb as I pulled out of the convenience store. He was underage but had a lot of cash laying around; I was twenty-one and had no qualms about committing what I assumed was a felony by buying my best friend a comically large amount of booze.

The idea was that if Four Loko, that wonderful, terrible metal tube of bright orange alcoholic juice bubbling with the potential energy of bad decisions, was made illegal, an underground market for its sale would flourish. Steve had been monitoring the news for weeks, hoping to figure out exactly when the public hysteria over the beverage would translate into some sort of policy change. And on this night, for whatever reason, it seemed that the other shoe was going to finally drop. He figured he could start selling the $3 cans at parties for 5 bucks a pop, raising the price point as his stash dwindled. When the announcement of the Great Decaffeination came soon thereafter, we celebrated Steve's imminent windfall by splitting a can and looking up rap songs about Four Loko on YouTube.

The story of the dumbest thing I ever did in college ended that Christmas Eve, when Steve was arrested for selling Four Loko to an undercover cop. He'd been hawking it on Craigslist, which he quickly learned was the sort of thing that law enforcement, for some reason, tends to find somewhat distasteful. Soon enough, he was sitting in the back of a squad car, giving directions to a friend's place, where the remainder of his stash lay waiting in the attic. Over the next thirty minutes, Steve and his arresting officers popped the top of every Loko he had left and poured them into a storm drain, a rainbow of profit running together to form a river of brown loss.

I never found out if what I did was a felony or not, because when the cops asked Steve where he got the goods, he lied and said he'd bought it all himself, and that the place hadn't checked his ID. Despite the implausibility of the story—who in their right minds *wouldn't* ask to see the ID of a college kid who was buying that much booze?—they took him at his word. The fact that it was Christmas Eve probably helped, if only because following up on his story would have been extra work and nobody wants to do that on Christmas Eve. But it didn't help Steve where his family was concerned. His parents had to skip Mass to bail him out, and when they all got home, his extremely Catholic mother collapsed on the floor and started saying Hail Marys.

Steve's fine these days, though. The entire case was so ridiculous that the judge nearly laughed him out of the courtroom and ended up sentencing him to probation. He went to grad school, got his PhD, and now is a college professor. We now live three blocks away from each other in Philadelphia, but for years we didn't live in the same city, so when we were together, we tried to make it count.

A few years ago, Steve was down in Durham visiting his parents when I texted him asking if he'd ever golfed before. *No*, he responded, *but fuck it*.

I took him to Twin Lakes, one of those old public courses that's never crowded (and was eventually, inevitably, sold to rapacious developers who built a housing development on it). Steve's hair goes down past his shoulders. He's built like an NFL linebacker and has flamboyantly bad taste in fashion. He has more energy than any other grown-up ever, and when he's not with his students, his default mode is exuberance.

His first attempt at a golf shot was a duffed drive; he immediately chased after the ball to hit it again, screaming, "Fuck you, golf!" He loved having no idea what he was doing, and I loved trying to explain it to him. Around the seventh hole, he figured out how to make perfect contact, and for the rest of the round he sporadically sent the ball astonishing distances. On the eighteenth hole, he hit such a good shot that, in triumph, he kicked in celebration and somehow managed to pop the tee marker up in the air, causing it to flip over and land spiky side out, and then he accidentally stomped on it, impaling his shoe upon the nail—which continued directly into his foot.

I asked him if he wanted me to drive him to the hospital, because that is what friends do. "Nah, dude, it's cool. Gotta see if I can get a par," he said, hobbling toward the green and three-putting for one of the more impressive bogeys I have ever encountered. He ended up having to get a tetanus booster, but besides that, he was fine.

Golf is a perfect vessel for getting together with people and sharing the feeling of being a kid again, because what is golf if not dressing up in the costume of "a Golfer" and playing with toys? As the years have passed, it's offered Steve and me the same sense of adventure that once caused us to enact a minor criminal conspiracy together.

The game brought us to Myrtle Beach in the early days of the pandemic, where we played a course made up of replicas of famous golf holes in the day and walked the city's main drag at night, gawking at the tens of thousands of tourists who wandered the street with drinks in hand as they went, maskless, into restaurants and bars; got pulled over for drunk-driving golf carts; and generally acted as if the coronavirus did not exist. Golf has taken us to a ritzy country club in the suburbs, where we played with a pair of grandmas who drove Teslas and called each other chickenshits when they left a putt short. One course we played featured a hole with a green guarded in the front by bunkers that rose out of the earth and sloped up to a highway, creating the shape of a miniature volcano. We each got caught in the trap and, one after the other, sent our balls sailing across the road. I went first and was able to run across the highway and pitch my ball back into play. Steve was less lucky, and he happened to hit his wayward shot at the very second a pickup truck was cruising past. His ball shattered its passenger-side rear window, shooting glass into the cab. The sound of a golf ball hitting a moving car window isn't a high-pitched cascade like it is in the movies. Instead, it's more of a dull thud, followed by profanity and screeching tires.

The guy wasn't exactly pissed off when he got out of the truck, because to call him pissed off would be to fundamentally misread the affect of the Southern, working-class male. Instead, when his boots touched pavement, he just sighed, as if he'd been driving past this course for years and figured this was going to happen one of these days. The dude riding shotgun stared straight down the road as Steve and the guy talked and I stood silent, blinking with anxiety and looking every which way. "This is gotta be about a five hunnerd dollar repair," the guy told Steve, and before Steve could respond, he said, "Well, actually, lemme call my buddy. He does body work, so maybe he'll know better'n me."

The good thing, the buddy told him, was that the window was broken clean off, so all he needed was a new window as opposed to having to pay somebody to dig a bunch of glass out of the suicide door panel, which meant it would be 150 bucks, tops. He agreed to meet us at a Sunoco off the highway on the way out of town so that Steve could give him the money, but when we showed up at the intersection he told us to go to, there were two Sunocos catty-corner from each other. Steve called the guy to ask which gas station he meant, but all he said was "Ah, whatever, I'm on the other side of town already," and he asked Steve to mail him a check when he had the chance. "I trust you," he told him. Steve followed through.

When Steve and I get together to golf, we're never worried about how we score. We take mulligans, goof off, and almost inevitably play so slowly that we end up having to let a few other groups play through. Most of the time, we go to a low-key course in the northern part of town, where one of us buys a six-pack of beer while the other pays the ridiculously low greens fee, and then we leisurely walk the course, oscillating between getting caught up on each other's lives, discussing the dense theory Steve studies, and talking massive amounts of smack. I'll razz him for his homegrown swing that occasionally leads him to either outdrive me or completely miss the ball; his digs tend to focus on the fact that I take golf way too seriously to be such an aggressively average player. But when one of us hits a genuinely great shot, there's nothing but effusive praise. And maybe just a *liiiiiitle* bit of shit-talking.

For better or (most definitely) for worse, as we get older and the organic connections of youth fade, many of us find ourselves reorienting our social lives around our careers. And as someone who was working remotely even before it was cool or strongly recommended by the government, I feel like I have some unique insight into this. Working in an actual space, whether it's a restaurant or an office or a store or whatever else, creates a nexus of shared experience, of genuine physical presence and camaraderie, that you just can't get from behind a screen. So much of sociality is based on proximity—noting an odd sideways glance, picking up on unspoken energies, developing a shared, mostly farcical enmity toward the guy in marketing who spends all day at his standing desk while shuffling atop a balance board. The place itself becomes a character in your world, offering routine while throwing the occasional curveball your way. And that, I think, is why I love golfing with my buddies so much. Even when the course is new, it's familiar enough to replicate the dynamic of the shared workspace, minus all the bad stuff—like actually having to work.

Then again, the golf course is also a bit of a playground for adults. You and your friends show up with your toys, then go out and play with them for a few hours. It's really that simple. Out there, your world becomes small again; life's challenges extend only to the out-of-bounds markers (or, in the case of Steve, slightly beyond them). And these are the ideal conditions for getting to know someone, even someone who's been in your life for years, better—together on the links, striving to succeed but liberated from the consequences of failure.

Chapter Seven

HOW GOLF MADE ME A BETTER LISTENER

NINE MONTHS INTO writing this book, I decided to take an inventory of how much I'd spent on golf since I'd begun. The amount was approximately $6,000. This included:

1. An average of $250 a month in greens fees at my local public course;
2. $100 every other month in greens fees at a different, very difficult course an hour away;
3. $170 for a used Titleist 815 D2 driver;
4. $625 for a new set of Cleveland UHX irons (four-iron through pitching wedge, originally $800 but discounted because I traded in some clubs);
5. $120 for a backup set of Mizuno MP-60 irons after I decided that I hated using the Clevelands;
6. $40 for a used Sonartec four-wood;

7. $160 a month for lessons from one of the top instructors in the state of North Carolina;
8. $75 for two boxes of premium golf balls ($40 for TaylorMade TP5x, $35 for Snell MTB Black);
9. $120 for two $60 pairs of Adidas golf shoes (one with spikes for maximum traction, one spikeless for maximum comfort when walking); and
10. $600 for a trip to Myrtle Beach, South Carolina, with my friend Steve, where we played two rounds of golf and drank so much beer that I threw up.

Looking at that number made me want to throw up again.

I told myself I would have spent some of that money on other things, leisure things if everything had been normal. But at the height of the pandemic, things were not normal, and my leisure activities were not plural. Maybe I can write it all off on my taxes or something.

The day I began writing this chapter, I shot an 82. That's 10 over par, a score that included seven pars, two birdies, five bogeys, four double bogeys, and five penalty strokes. On the back nine, I shot a 39, an achievement unto itself. Prior to my flurry of golf investing, I had shot less than 40 on nine holes only once, when I was a junior in high school. I spent $6,000 to get to where I had a reasonable chance of doing so every time I stepped on my home course.

Actually, I should say $6,060, because now that I think of it, I spent $60 on a premium subscription to an app called V1 Game, which tracks every shot I hit during every round of golf I play. Looking at it now, it's showing me that if I hadn't notched those penalty strokes, had been a bit less sloppy around the greens, and had made a few more easy putts, I would have shot even par. This is nice to know. It's knowledge like this—the feeling that I'm getting better all the time, and I can see all the ways in which I can make my scores match how I'm feeling—that turned playing golf into a compulsion.

• • •

I once read an article in an anarchist zine that claimed golf was the sport that was most "of the earth." Something to do with how the motion of swinging a club is kind of like sweeping the grass, giving it a little haircut, treating the earth not as a subject to be dominated but a collaborator in a project that's greater than either of you, etc. I like the sentiment, but I'm not sure whoever wrote it actually played golf. Sometimes, nature becomes the enemy. Sometimes, you are your own enemy.

Just before twilight one evening, I played seven holes with my golf teacher, a soft-spoken man named Jimmy Hamilton who has played in multiple Champions Tour events. I'd been taking lessons from him for months, and under his tutelage I'd completely reworked my swing from an ungainly, homegrown whirl of limbs into something respectable-looking, which, at least when Jimmy was watching, allowed me to be consistent within the controlled confines of the driving range. On the course, not so much: I got three pars and three double bogeys, and picked up prior to reaching the green on the final hole out of frustration.

"It's like I was two different golfers, only one of whom knew what they were doing," I said as he drove our golf cart to the parking lot.

"No, this was good," he told me. "Now I know what we need to work on." His coaching style involved watching me hit balls, coming up with the what-to-do, how-to-do-it, and why-you-should-do-it of a swing change, telling me two of them, and leaving me to figure out the third. On the course, he kept telling me to maintain my tempo and balance, because I was swinging so fast it looked like I was on the verge of falling over. Playing good golf is about lots of things—thinking critically about how each shot will set up the next and making your club selections accordingly, being creative with greenside shots, and developing feel with your putter. But without tempo and control over your body, those things don't really mean anything, because the ball won't go where you want it to, and by the time the wedges come into play, you're chipping for bogey or worse. This was not an isolated incident.

After Jimmy had given me a new swing, I gave myself new problems. Specifically: My tempo was killing me. As I made my way through a round, I started swinging faster and faster, which is half of what you're supposed to do. You want to go back slowly, winding your arms and torso and legs until you get to the point where you've "loaded the shaft"—a term I couldn't really explain verbally, but which I could feel when I did it properly—and then let yourself swing fast on the way through. Executed successfully, the whole thing is like pulling a rubber band back on your finger and then shooting it across the room.

But it's a matter of *letting* yourself swing fast, not *doing* a fast swing. Whenever I had a few good holes, the adrenaline kicked in and told me to start swinging hard. I began to bring the club back too quickly, which sent me off-balance. This is a thing that happens because golf clubs are sticks with weights at the end, comparable-ish in function to the stick you hold while walking the tightrope, except instead of using it to maintain your balance while walking, you use it to maintain your balance while swinging it, in a way that leads to the middle part of the clubface striking the golf ball. I think this is part of the reason golfers complain they're better on the driving range than on the course—during a round, you're walking without a net.

• • •

In the mornings, I wrote my book about golf. In the afternoons, I went to the golf course and played. After I shot the 82, the bottom fell out of my game. I couldn't get under the ball to save my life. Instead, I sent shot after shot skittering on the ground—or at best, thirty feet in the air, which meant that rather than having high, arcing shots coming to a soft rest wherever they landed, these were line drives that rolled out unpredictably, sometimes way past where they ought to be and, on wet days, unceremoniously plopping into the soggy ground well short of my target. As my scores went up and my shots stayed down and nothing I did seemed to change anything, I began to feel like the guy in Greek mythology who pissed off the gods and was damned to have his liver pecked out by some bird, only to have it grow back so the whole process could play itself out again the next day. Prometheus?

I just googled it, and it's definitely Prometheus.

"You're in your own head, dude," my friend Charlie, the one who sold me the four-wood, told me. We were on the second-to-last hole of his country club, and I was about to shoot my worst score in probably three years. The course was hard, so I'd practiced for an hour before going there, trying to smooth out the jerky tempo that I suspected was to blame for my recent inconsistency. After a hundred balls or so, I got everything grooved, but it was too much preparation for walking eighteen holes. I tired out almost immediately, my muscles misremembering the rhythm and sequence.

Every shot seemed to be the wrong one, and I felt lucky to make even a bogey. Every time I thought I'd overcome whatever had gotten into me, I'd flub a drive, skull a chip, or overcorrect my hook, only to start slicing. Another self-directed insult added to self-inflicted injury arrived after I knocked a pretty great three-wood off the tee and left myself with an uphill approach to the green. I hit my seven-iron about as perfectly as I'd been able to all day, high and straight and beautiful and listing right just enough to hold the green once it landed—only it was the wrong club, and I ended up ten yards short, just behind a bunker, which I needed to chip over to even think about saving par.

Emotions, specifically mine, were high, and I had sweated sunscreen into my eye. It stung, and I couldn't tell if Charlie thought I was crying or not.

"Hit another one," he said. He's a good friend and an even better person, and the kindness with which he offered this suggestion definitely implied that he thought I was crying. After we finished, I asked Charlie to scratch my round out on the scorecard instead of adding it all up. I didn't want to think about how I'd played that day, and I definitely didn't want to write about it.

But this is how golf works. In order to get better, you have to bottom out; otherwise, you won't know what to fix.

• • •

For my next lesson, Jimmy the golf teacher had me do an exercise where I swung slowly, putting all my weight on my back foot so that I could feel my torso coil before letting go. He said this would help my tempo but left the why blank this time. It worked perfectly on the driving range and then exploded in my face when I attempted to replicate it alone on the course, suddenly bereft of his encouragement when I'd get it right, as well as his corrections for when I got it wrong. Only after I gave up on being perfect did I understand the why behind it all: You exaggerate the swing change knowing that you will go back to normal. Or at least that's what you perceive. Because the exercise stays with you. It *felt* like nothing had changed, but I could tell that my swing had gotten a little easier, my balance a little more stable, and I approached every swing with a newfound sense of control.

One day, I shot 83. This time, my best shots didn't go as far, but my worst shots didn't destroy my sense of self. This is progress. Driving home, I thought about how high my scores had been the previous year compared with where I was that day, even when I took my extended blowup period into account. Over the next few weeks, I stayed in the mid- to low-80s, about seven or so strokes lower than where I'd once been. The run of bad scores I'd been having were outliers. Too often in life, it's the outliers we focus on. But if we zoom out and look at the big picture, we see that often everything deviates to the mean.

My golf teacher once told me that the best athletes have short-term memory problems. If they screw up, it rolls off their backs. If they do something amazing, it does not, cannot, affect what they're about to do next, either. The rest of us, our errors compound while our successes become burdens.

When I was a high school soccer player, I was named an all-conference goalkeeper. I mainly succeeded because the kids I played with were so good that they made it nearly impossible for the other team to get off a solid shot, though I once made the local news for blocking two penalty kicks in a single game against one of the best teams in the state. My senior year, we ended up going all the way to the state championship. About a third of the way through the game, our center midfielder placed a shot in the top right corner of the net to put us one up. Minutes later, the other team kicked a high cross toward the goal with the hope that one of their guys would knock it in with his head. There wasn't anybody else around, so I was the only person who was going to be able to make that not happen. I jumped high, swinging my right leg up like I was walking up some stairs so I could protect my body while rotating toward the ball. The player who was closest to me dove toward where the ball was supposed to be, but my hip was there instead.

There was a crack.

An ambulance arrived. The whole thing got his teammates so amped up that they came back and nearly blew us off the field. It was like I was letting them score out of guilt. Maybe I was. The kid ended up being fine and made it back to the sidelines in time to catch the final whistle and get hoisted up by his teammates in celebration. It was very inspiring. I've hated competition ever since.

• • •

Jimmy decided that he would teach me about putting. "Seems easy enough," I joked as we made our way to the practice green.

"Easy to screw up," he said.

He set me up about ten feet away from the cup and told me to have at it. I'd never really thought about the way I putted before; it was just a thing that I did, really. You sit behind the ball and check the contours of the green, pick a line you judge most likely to account for the break, get up, take the putter back, and then hopefully something good happens. Jimmy watched as I sent a couple of balls into the cup; most ended up around it, and a few blew past it, catching the slope of the green and rolling toward some high school kids.

He smiled one of those smiles that's not really a smile. "Lemme check something," he said. "Hold your putter again."

I stood with my putter—a big, silly red thing that looked a little bit like a race car but was called a Spider—how I normally did: my hands wrapped around the very bottom of its synthetic leather grip, the ball directly between my legs, my shoulders so hunched that an onlooker with a healthy imagination might have worried they were being absorbed by my chest.

"You don't look very natural," Jimmy said. He whistled. "I think your putter's too long for your arms."

He went to his bag and grabbed his own, much shorter putter. "Try this," he said. "And have the ball below your left eye," he added. "Looks like you favor it."

It turned out that because the ball wasn't below my dominant eye, I was misjudging it, and because my putter was too long, I was standing too far away from it, creating a weird angle between its face and the ground. With a shorter putter in my hands, counterintuitively enough, I no longer slumped over, instead standing tall and balanced, confidently letting the putter glide in a short, sweet arc. The putts started going in. It was as if my body had known how to play the song all along, but I'd given it the wrong instrument. I had a shorter putter in my trunk; I switched over to it the next round after the lesson and didn't look back.

The next week, Jimmy gave me a lesson in chipping. "Grab your wedges, plus your nine-iron and your eight-iron," he told me.

We met at the short game area, the least used yet most important part of any self-respecting golf practice facility. For many golfers, including me, a well-placed chip or pitch can be the difference between par and double bogey. The fact of the matter is that swinging a golf club really fast and making the exact center of its face hit a little golf ball is ridiculously hard. Most people hit only a few perfect shots during a round.

"You gotta make it up somewhere," Jimmy said. "If you young guys practiced chipping as much as you did hitting your drivers, all y'all'd be on Tour by now." This was flattering to hear, even if both Jimmy and I knew that I was not going to make any tour, ever, except for a guided one through a museum. He was right. In the fifteen years or so since I'd last had a golf lesson, I'd all but forgotten how to hit a proper short shot; when I was within fifty or so yards of the green, I'd just grab my lob wedge and artlessly slap at the ball in the hope that I'd end up closer to the hole than I had been. Sometimes, I'd have to do this twice, though, or even three times. It was not, strictly speaking, ideal.

"Every wedge is a tool," Jimmy explained, "and you use each of 'em the same way." By this, he meant that there are really only two shots to the short game: the low one and the high one. The low ones are meant to be a putt, basically. Jimmy had me set up holding my pitching wedge about ten feet away from the green, leaning forward while the ball rested in my stance toward my back toe, my hands resting so that the club's shaft leaned forward. This was to decrease the angle made between my pitching wedge and the ground, he explained, because what I was learning to do was essentially a putt, but one that began with a pop off the ground in order to clear all the shaggy grass guarding the green's smooth surface. "Pick a spot on the green where you want it to start rolling at, and aim there," he said.

You hit the low bump-and-run shot with the same gentle rocking of the arms no matter how much real estate you've got to cover, he told me; if the cup's farther away, you do the same thing but use a club with lower loft, such as a seven-iron. "Easiest shot in the world," Jimmy told me. After a few cracks at it from a few different spots, I was inclined to agree.

"But what about if I've got, like, ten feet before the green and then the pin is right there?" I asked. I knew the answer to this was that I was going to have to hit the high shot, but I asked anyway because I wanted him to teach me how to pull it off. One of the biggest challenges with short, arcing pitch shots is that in order to make it go high, you've got to get your wedge down into the ground so that it can get under the ball. But I'd always been jumpy whenever I'd try one of these, and instead would attempt to lift the ball up in the air with my wedge, often causing me to just smack the ball with the edge of the club, yielding a line drive that skittered past my target.

The secret, Jimmy showed me, wasn't a secret at all. The high shot is just the inverse of the low shot. Ball toward your front foot, face of the wedge slightly open, hands leaning slightly toward your belt buckle. "That's called engaging the bounce," he said. By that, he meant that every clubhead creates an angle against the ground that is meant to help it glide over the turf. Wedges have a lot of bounce, which allows you to drive them downward and keep them there as they slide under the ball. The less room your ball has to roll, the higher the loft of wedge you should use. "The key to this one is to commit," he said, "because you're gonna be making a swing that feels too big for how short it's gonna go. But just keep it nice and slow, and the ball'll do what it should."

Lob wedge with fifteen feet to the pin: pop, pop, pop, pop, all ending up within ten feet of the pin—the kind of distance that gave me a fighting chance of sinking it with one putt. Same thing with the sand wedge from twenty and the gap wedge from thirty. "Don't use the lob wedge too much," he said. "The simplest path to the hole is the best one. Just make sure you've got the right tool, and you'll be fine."

• • •

Golf clubs are kind of like cars in that they should really last you about twenty years, but lots of people buy new ones every year anyway. When I started the job I was eventually laid off from, I immediately went out and bought a convertible. A cheap one—an old Volkswagen Cabrio with no cruise control and a leaky top—but a convertible nonetheless. I drove it all summer, top down, and eventually the heat and humidity caused so much damage to the CD player that it managed to fuse with my copy of *The Best of Motörhead*, which had been living inside of it.

I didn't know that you're supposed to drive old cars once a week to keep the battery running properly, and by the time I got laid off the next spring, the battery in the Cabrio was dead and so was the rest of the car.

Let's add $200 to the $6,060 I've spent on golf, because I just bought yet another driver, this one a Callaway Mavrik Max. I now own five drivers, six fairway woods, five hybrids, three sets of irons (one containing six clubs; another seven, and the third eight), seven wedges, and six putters. This means I own forty-nine golf clubs. The rules of golf say you can carry fourteen of them during a round. Most of them I bought cheap, usually at thrift stores, and fiddled around with them for a couple of rounds before inevitably returning to my normal set, ultimately letting my new old clubs take up space in our living room, leaning up in a corner behind a fake fireplace that my gullible step-grandmother, God love her, swore was handcrafted by the Amish. I keep them all, I tell myself, because I need them. I keep a full backup set in case anything ever happens to my own clubs, plus another that I lend to friends when I take them golfing. I definitely don't need six putters; it would be more reasonable to keep three: the one I actually use; another one that's a different style in case I want to change; and the last one, a vintage hickory-shafted model, to frame and hang on the wall. Same with the wedges and hybrids and woods: Keep one backup, turn the really old ones into decorations, and sell or donate everything else.

The problem is that, like cars, every golf club is slightly different, and they're all worth different amounts. The more a club is worth, the more I would convince myself that I should keep it just in case. With the ones that weren't worth anything, I'd say, there's not really a point to getting rid of them. And so they collected dust, slowly transforming the corner of our living room into a garage full of undriven cars with dead batteries, and, by osmosis, me into the middle-aged divorced dad who discovered that a convertible didn't fit into the hole in his heart only after it was already too late. At least that guy knows why he does the pointless things he does. His reasons are all sad ones, but they're reasons nonetheless.

• • •

Oh! I meant to tell you this earlier: Golf isn't really about competition. It's about remaining calm and allowing yourself to play golf.

Jimmy taught me that. When I started playing with my new driver, it felt weird. It was too light. I couldn't swing as hard as I wanted, because when I did, the ball would fly in any direction other than straight. Jimmy always told me I swung too hard, but I could never figure out how not to: I had to swing hard with my old driver, or else it wouldn't go. But that made me start swinging every other club hard, too, and then that made the ball do unfortunate and funky stuff. I'd go to the driving range and try everything, messing with where I set my feet, how I brought the club back, the angle of my right elbow, my posture. It all helped for a moment, but as long as I was swinging hard, my muscles didn't stand a chance of keeping it all in sequence for too long.

After the 83, the beautiful, glorious 83, my scores crept back up. The what was that I needed to get more consistent. The why was self-evident. The how was trickier, or at least I thought so until I realized this: It all goes back to the tempo. Fiddling with my new driver on the range, I tried Jimmy's all-the-weight-on-the-back-foot exercise again, taking the time to really feel what I was doing. I began to notice that when I took my arms back, there was a point at which they sort of stopped, just naturally so, and if I let them do it, I could feel my hips and chest and shoulders turn, my muscles tensing together in sync as if to signal they were ready to come down and hit the ball. And when I let it happen, the ball flew and flew, so effortlessly that I was sure that swinging this way was somehow cheating. Jimmy hadn't been telling me to swing more slowly, even if those were the words he used. He was telling me to listen to my club, which was telling me to listen to my body, which was telling me it wanted to stop my backswing at this point of perfect synchronization, and I'd have realized it all sooner if I hadn't been blowing through this delicate moment like a drunk driver at a four-way stop.

Jimmy had been trying, for months, to say that a golf club wants to go however fast it's going to go, and that forcing it was a fool's errand. You can't just tell that to somebody, though. You can't really tell people anything. You have to let them realize it for themselves, and for Jimmy, that meant having the demeanor of a therapist and the corresponding patience of a saint, allowing clients to screw up over and over again but always encouraging, always prodding in the right direction, blowing the exact right amount of information into their sails so that once they get everything calibrated on their end, they don't need your help steering the ship.

Chapter Eight

HOW GOLF TAUGHT ME TO KEEP FIGHTING THE GOOD FIGHT

AMERICA IS FULL of inequality, and that's by design. I don't mean designed by the machinations of a group of shady power brokers in smoke-filled rooms or alien lizard people. It's more like America is a machine whose gears have slid and rearranged themselves, often intentionally, over time, until it began to produce certain outcomes, namely those favoring the rich and powerful and white, simply through force of precedence. But the rich and powerful like the results the machine spits out, and they're willing to do damn near anything they have to in order to convince us all that despite all the steam and creaks and groans coming out of it, the machine is doing great thank you very much and we definitely don't need to fix it at all. In fact, this machine isn't a machine at all and is instead simply the natural order of things, or maybe if it is a machine, and by no means are we saying it is one, then it was here before we were and it's so big that we could never so much as dream of disassembling it.

Life is hard, and it's easy to get caught up trying to not go broke that we end up not noticing who's getting richer off our misery.

Similarly, we can divide golfers into two groups: those who regularly play on expensive courses, and golfers who can't afford to do that. And honestly, fancy golf courses are great. They're less crowded, the fairways are immaculately manicured, there's soft sand in every bunker, and every green rolls true. I've always considered myself a member of the sport's middle class, spending most of my time knocking around my local muni and occasionally shelling out $100 or so for a round on a primo track. But that's a facile take on my own situation: If I spend $100 on golf one day, that's $100 I will have to forgo spending on something else. There are people in this world who do not face such binary choices.

"Class" is a tricky concept, often tied up in notions such as taste, education, manners, accent, and a general air of worldliness. But really, the main marker of distinction is money. The rest of that stuff makes you appear to be of a certain class, but money can buy the rest of that stuff. And if you rise to wealth from nothing and can't fake it or don't want to, just give it a generation or two. What was unnatural to you becomes water to your progeny.

All good golf movies, I'm convinced, are about class. This is an easy claim to make, because in my mind there are only two good golf movies, and they are *Caddyshack* and *Happy Gilmore*. At their core, each film is about outsiders sticking a finger in the eye of exclusive communities, composed of people who keep the ranks closed by affecting a sense of stuffy refinement. Al Czervik, Rodney Dangerfield's louche, wisecracking windbag, is effectively the protagonist of *Caddyshack*, driving the plot through his actions and spending much of his time onscreen antagonizing the other members of Bushwood Country Club while forging a camaraderie with the caddies and the other working stiffs just trying to hold their noses in front of the rich assholes long enough to make a few bucks and go home. While Judge Smails, the film's villain who haughtily rules the country club with an iron fist, tells the main caddy, Danny, that he's "sentenced boys younger than you to the gas chamber" because he "owed it to them," Czervik's throwing money around to those who don't have it and later joining forces with the underdog Danny and the affable, affluent New Ager Ty Webb.

Happy Gilmore, meanwhile, is part of a lineage of doofy mainstream American films accidentally indebted to the low-stakes, high-pressure, working-class struggle perfected by Vittorio De Sica's *Bicycle Thieves* (see also *The Warriors*, *Rudy*, and *8 Mile*). Literally the only reason that Adam Sandler's title character becomes a professional golfer is that he needs money in order to rescue his grandmother from a nursing home, where she's being tortured by Ben Stiller's mustachioed Nurse Ratched–style orderly. Happy figures out how to hit the ball a billion miles using decrepit clubs while injecting a rowdiness into the pro tour, infuriating the competition with his casual attitude and penchant for getting into fistfights with Bob Barker. That Happy wins with the help of a Black coach, Chubbs Peterson—a former champion who gets rejected from the sport's inner sanctum after losing his hand in an unfortunate incident involving an alligator—feels apt: Through Happy's success, Chubbs can claim his revenge. *Happy Gilmore* may not have intentionally created a model of Black-white working-class solidarity on purpose, but sometimes you've got to separate the art from the artist.

But most people with money aren't good-vibes Robin Hoods like Al in *Caddyshack*, and most broke golfers don't have Happy's innate ability to hit the hell out of a golf ball. Because those are movie characters, it's narratively expedient for them to kick in the establishment's metaphorical door. But in real life, there's rarely a door at all: Instead, there's a ladder, which most people pull up behind them once scaled.

I thought about all of this one day while sitting in the parking lot of Pinehurst, the legendary North Carolina golf resort, waiting to meet my dad for a round of golf at Pinehurst No. 2, the most storied—and expensive—of the compound's nine championship-level golf courses. It was around the start of summer 2020, and the round was my dad's way of saying, "Sorry you got laid off." He hoped playing Pinehurst would take my mind off things, and besides, I'd begun thinking of writing a book on golf (namely, this one), and he figured the round might inspire something.

It was the Trump bumper stickers around me, I think, that really got my brain working overtime: TRUMP 2020, KEEP AMERICA GREAT, TRUMP 2020 NO MORE BULLSHIT—all the hits. They were on BMW X5s, on Ford F-150s, on sports cars designed to look constantly in motion, so full of angles and curves that it was a wonder they had enough flat space for a bumper sticker at all. This is what I mean when I say that class is about money more than taste: These pieces of mechanical perfection beg to be ogled by all, asking us to marvel at their comfort, their speed, their power; they are advertisements for the wealth of those who drive them, and their stickers are advertisements for how few fucks those drivers truly give. They say, "Not only do I have this fancy motorized toy and you don't, but I vote in a way that will make it harder for you to *ever* have a toy like this."

• • •

Founded in 1895 by James Walker Tufts, Pinehurst was originally a healthful getaway for those suffering from tuberculosis—the freshness of the North Carolina air, it was thought, could reinvigorate the lungs. Tufts, who'd done quite well for himself in the soda fountain business, enlisted the expertise of Frederick Law Olmsted, the landscape architect behind New York's Central Park and Prospect Park, to lay out the grounds. In 1898, the first course was set up; three years later, a young pro named Donald Ross was brought in to oversee the golf side of the operation, which quickly became the resort's main focus, overtaking its initial priority of rest and rejuvenation. Ross had previously been apprenticed to Old Tom Morris, the head golf professional at St. Andrews who was also responsible for many of the most iconic links courses in Scotland, and in the area's unique mix of windswept sand and pine forests, Ross found the ideal canvas for translating Scottish design principles onto American terrain. He renovated Pinehurst's course, doing such a good job that they let him throw in two more for the hell of it. The first of them, Pinehurst No. 2, opened in 1907. With its tight fairways, endless stretches of waste bunkers, and bedeviling greens, whose quick speeds and subtle angles can send a misstruck putt back onto the fairway, remains one of the most psychotically difficult golf courses in existence.

No. 2 put Pinehurst on the map, almost immediately establishing the course as one of the finest tests of golfing ability in the nation, attracting a robust community of wealthy golfers looking to spend winters away from the cold industrial hellhole they had to put up with in order to oversee their dad's factory or whatever. Today, Pinehurst boasts nine full courses, a par 3 course called the Cradle, croquet grounds, five lodging options, a spa, ten restaurants, miles of trails, a two-hundred-acre lake, the museum-like Tufts Archives, complimentary use of BMWs for guests interested in taking a self-guided driving tour around the area, and a staff of more than thirteen hundred who, if it's their job to greet you by phone or in person, do so by saying, "It's a beautiful day in Pinehurst." Needless to say, they are never lying.

The beautiful day that my dad and I played there, it was three weeks into nationwide protests in response to the murder of George Floyd by members of the Minneapolis Police Department; the protests had started in the Twin Cities and within hours spread throughout the country as more police departments attempted to put out the fire of dissent with the gasoline of violent repression. The night before I met my dad for a round, my partner and I had attended a protest in downtown Durham, then gone home and watched as a correspondent from the anarchist news collective Unicorn Riot livestreamed a group of people breaking into a Minneapolis precinct and setting it ablaze. "It's a beautiful day in Pinehurst," joked a guy in a pink polo to his friend as they walked past me warming up on the putting green, "'cuz there ain't no fuckin' riots here!" I suddenly felt like an unwanted infiltrator, or perhaps a spy. For whom, I wasn't quite sure.

• • •

One of the reasons some people hate journalists is that we have the unique ability to broadcast people's lowest moments. When they're talking to us and they say or do something they shouldn't, it is literally our job to tell everyone about it. We find out the things you wish were private and make them public. We dig through public records, connect dots, ask around about who knows what. Any journalists with a sense of ethics deploy their arsenal primarily to hold the powerful to account. If you're a CEO who claims to care about the environment but dumps toxic waste onto baby goat farms for fun, we'll tell the world about it. If you're just some rando who's had a terrible day and insults a stranger out of frustration, not so much.

But people don't necessarily realize this, and it makes sense. Most of the time, news stories become part of the public conversation only when they unearth that someone or some entity has done something wild. The presidency of Donald Trump was an exception to this, because he did so much fascinating, repulsive, and downright crazy stuff that even people who hated him followed his every move. So, to a certain degree, it's natural that lots of people would assume that every journalist's job is to dig up dirt on everyone, and pore over people's entire lives with a fine-tooth comb in order to assemble the least flattering portrait of them possible. And it's especially likely if they perceive a journalist as having a well-defined view of the world, especially one that they think is misaligned with their own.

The things I care about, not to mention write about, are often in direct opposition to golf, or at least golf as people tend to conceive of it. Expensive golf courses are expensive because they're trying to keep people *out*, which I believe is unfair on a fundamental level. The reason a slogan like "Abolish the police" is so threatening and strange to people like the ones I overheard at Pinehurst is that at Pinehurst and places like it, the police basically don't exist. The cops would never search someone's car for drugs here, or shoot someone in cold blood for shoplifting a sleeve of balls from the pro shop, because our society assumes that if you're at a place like Pinehurst as a paying customer, then you must have money, and therefore you belong. The police exist to protect those who belong from those who don't.

But this is the way America works. This version of golf is part of a larger system in which the many watch helplessly as what little they have is slowly siphoned off by the few. Student loans, credit card debt, car payments, rent, pharmaceutical and medical bills, for-profit prisons and rehab centers, retirement communities, wage stagnation, layoffs to boost margins on a quarterly earnings report, the funneling of labor from salaried work into the gig economy, private equity firms, the financialization of debt, the elimination of small businesses and the opportunities to start them, you name it—all of this makes money flow one way, and it's probably not toward you or me. The margins by which the winners win and the losers lose tend to compound, making it so that if you lose even once, you'll have a worse chance of winning, especially without cheating, for the rest of your life.

And the winners can afford to do things like pay as much as $500 to play a round at Pinehurst, or even join—it costs a minimum of $25,000 *plus* a monthly fee to even have discounted rates here, a figure that jumps up to $45,000 upfront and $620 a month for unfettered access. Technically, the cheapest way to join Pinehurst is to buy a home that carries with it a preexisting membership; go about it this way, and you pay half price to transfer it to your name. So, in order to get the best deal, you've got to spend the most money. It's a great deal for those who already have a membership, because it turns those memberships into assets to be bought and sold, a neat way to boost the property value of the homes they are attached to. This reveals a fundamental truth about America: We love the possibility of success, these markers of status, so much so that we sometimes don't bother to look at the strings attached. And we certainly don't follow those strings until we make our way to whoever's holding them, ready to tug our hopes and dreams away at the exact moment when it seems they may just become real.

• • •

Pinehurst was great, by the way. I shot a 52 on the front, thanks to multiple putts that I accidentally sent off the green, but I ended up with a 45 on the back—averaging a bogey a hole, basically—once I finally figured out how to putt on the damn greens. Coming up the eighteenth fairway to the final green, we saw a group of older women sitting on the clubhouse's veranda, drinking something fancy and serving as an impromptu gallery like they have at real golf tournaments. My dad made a twenty-five-foot putt for par to close everything out, and the ladies lost it. Loved Pinehurst, 10/10.

That's for the course itself. Pinehurst the institution definitely loses points for its insanely exclusive nature, its cultish devotion to its own mythology, and probably the personalities of maybe half the people who happened to be hanging out while I was there.

Besides being difficult to the point of tenacity, the biggest impression that No. 2 left with me was the very self-conscious way in which it presented itself as a piece of living history. The caddies functioned almost like tour guides, pointing out this seemingly arbitrary bump in the fairway or that waste bunker spanning the length of the hole and expounding upon how it reflected the original vision of Donald Ross, whose name was never uttered in tones anything less than hallowed. Smack-dab between the practice tee, the eighteenth green, and the clubhouse are four statues: Ross; Tufts; the late Payne Stewart, who dramatically won the U.S. Open there in 1999, just a few months before he died in a plane crash; and Robert H. Dedman, whose company Clubcorp gave new life to Pinehurst in a time of late twentieth-century economic distress. As one of our caddies showed them to us, we noticed that a bird had crapped upon Dedman's head. The caddy shrugged.

More history: In December 1912, a guy named Robert Hunter walked onto Pinehurst No. 2 and defeated Walter Travis, a three-time U.S. Amateur winner who'd notched the lowest score for an amateur at the U.S. Open just months earlier. Travis was, at the time, likely the winningest amateur in American match play history, a man who lived and breathed the game. He wrote numerous books and articles on golf, founded and published the *American Golfer* magazine, and worked to design and renovate golf courses himself. Here was someone who was a golf professional even if he was not technically a professional golfer, and he'd just gotten beat by Robert Hunter, who was just some guy.

To be clear, calling Robert Hunter "just some guy" downplays how unlikely it was that he'd be stepping foot upon Pinehurst at all, let alone winning golf tournaments there. Hunter was, at the time, one of the most well-known members of the Socialist Party of America, alongside the likes of authors Jack London and Upton Sinclair, perennial presidential contender Eugene V. Debs, and Representative Victor L. Berger. Four years prior, Hunter had been accused of giving a speech in New York City's Union Square that, according to a *New York Times* editorial, "implant[ed] ideas subversive of law and justice and order" into a crowd and led to somebody setting off a bomb. He was a pen pal of Leo Tolstoy; had been a delegate at the 1907 Second International Socialist Congress, attending alongside the likes of Rosa Luxemburg, George

Bernard Shaw, and Vladimir Lenin (he thought Lenin was secretly a cop); and had made his name advocating for then-radical policies such as social security for the old, women's suffrage, equal rights for all races, free school lunches for the young, and a minimum wage for all. On top of that, Hunter spent vast amounts of time at Pinehurst, competing in tournaments, joining a sporting society down there, and making the place his home away from home. I wonder if he felt like a spy, too.

I first came across Robert Hunter while researching golf books, trying to map out some of the texts that had been foundational to the conceptualization of the game in America. I learned that Hunter, in 1926, wrote a book called *The Links*, which was meant to serve as a how-to manual for aspiring golf course architects. By that point, Hunter had become friendly with nearly all the top course designers of the day, and he used *The Links* to pass on their tips, diagrams, and philosophies. The book functions both as a manual for how to design a golf course and as a treatise on what makes them work on both a practical and philosophical level.

During the plum years between World War I and the Great Depression, golf was gaining in popularity. The reforms that Hunter and his comrades had fought for had started to take hold, and working people had more free time than ever before. "Golf has been taken to the heart of Demos," Hunter wrote, prophesizing that "the time seems not far distant when every man, woman, and child will have a set of clubs." Public golf courses were on the rise, and Hunter's book presented itself as a field guide for nonprofessionals who'd suddenly been conscripted into designing their new public golf course, with the ultimate goal that "the immense sums now flowing into golf" could be "used to mould all over this country lovely landscapes to refresh the soul."

Hunter liked courses that made minimal changes to the landscape, thought that hazards like sand traps and ponds should be placed in a way that inspired golfers to be creative rather than penalized them for screwing up, and prized the quality of care given to a course over all else, to the point that he thought a course with five nicely manicured holes was automatically better than some eighteen-hole goat track. In his eyes, if a person could design a cheap municipal course that challenged golfers and brought out the best in their game, then that course could serve as a social equalizer, providing a space where everyone, both the privileged and working class, could meet—and would want to meet—and play together.

I sometimes worry that being a golfer with radical politics carries with it a certain set of contradictions, or that my love of golf makes me a bad socialist. Like, if I want to play the best courses, I have to shell out money I normally don't have, yet I do it anyway. Does this make me a willing participant in a system that takes us away from a more equitable world? Will people take me seriously when I talk about the problems of capitalism if I'm obsessed with a sport that most people perceive as being only for the rich?

To Hunter, there was no such contradiction; everyone deserved the good life. In fact, his embrace of golf helped get him into the mental space where he was able to get his message out. So let's rewind a moment and tell the story of Robert Hunter's life. Cue the wiggly screen and the do-do-do-doot sounds a là *Wayne's World*.

Robert Hunter was born in 1874 in Terre Haute, Indiana, the son of a well-to-do manufacturer of horse-drawn carriages and Civil War veteran on the Union side. After graduating from Indiana University, he trucked it out to Chicago, where he lived in Hull House, the famous experimental community dedicated to social reform founded by Jane Addams. If you'd grown up moneyed and sheltered, working-class Chicago was gross and sort of terrifying; Hunter later wrote of visiting a flophouse in the city and recoiling in horror at men sleeping on newspaper-covered floors, using their coats as pillows, others packed onto shelves that had been repurposed as beds, and a child sleeping on an upturned box because he was afraid of all the rats running around the place. "I made a thorough search for a place to sleep, but, not being successful in finding an unoccupied spot, I decided not to remain for the night," he wrote. "The air made me faint and weak, and I hardly had strength to pick my way out of the room."

It was during this time that Hunter came upon the same realization that lots of rich kids do once they make their way into the world: There are people whose lives are truly terrible due to no fault of their own, and you can choose to ignore the problem, gloat about it like an asshole, or try to do something about it. Hunter went with option three, to an almost self-parodic degree. He and his wife, the reformist-minded heiress Caroline Stokes, moved to Greenwich Village in New York, where they could be close to the city's working-class and immigrant populations, enacting what was, depending on the source, literally or figuratively an open-door policy in their home so that they could help whoever, however, whenever. Hunter gave away every coat he had to the homeless, and instead of replacing his own, he opted to shiver in solidarity for the entire winter as some sort of personal endurance test or example of Christlike sacrifice. Drawing from his experiences in both Chicago and New York, as well as mounds of statistics, charts, and tables, in 1903 Hunter began putting together a book on poverty called, uh, *Poverty*.

Published the next year, *Poverty* hit like a bomb (a metaphorical one, rather than the actual bomb that he did *not* cause to be set off in 1908). It described a world in which employment was precarious, yet simply hanging out and not working could be punished by jail time, where 1 percent of America owned 54.8 percent of its wealth, where few owned their own homes, and where wages were so low that even many who had jobs still couldn't get by. He viewed poverty as a "suction force," easy to slip into but hard to escape, and proposed that America institute a social safety net including unemployment insurance, workers' compensation, the decriminalization of addiction, and a system that we would now recognize as Social Security. "We put property before human life," he wrote indignantly. "We unconsciously estimate it more highly and foster it more tenderly; we do it as individuals and we do it collectively."

But Hunter worked so hard on *Poverty* that it nearly did him in. From what I found on him, he didn't seem like a very strong dude physically. A 1905 *New York Times* profile describes an early thirties Hunter as "spare of face and figure, with brown hair gradually retreating from an exceptionally high forehead," while also making note of his "well-shaped feet." Eventually, all this researching and writing and moralizing and shivering caused Hunter to have something of a nervous breakdown, and his doctor sent him and his wife packing for the countryside and told him to do more physical exercise. So Robert Hunter took up golf, writing in the mornings before hitting the links with a local pro in the afternoons. Before long, he struck up a golfing friendship with Finley Peter Dunne, the humorist famous for his fictional character Mr. Dooley, an Irish bartender in Chicago; in his memoirs, Hunter also recalled having played with the department store magnate Marshall Field as well as the muckraking journalist Lincoln Steffens. Competitively, Hunter went toe to toe with some of the best golfers, professional and amateur, in the country, once even beating the noted Scottish professional Stewart Gardner in match play.

One of the qualities of history, as with literature, is that we occasionally find pieces of ourselves within others. How many of us have come to the game at a time of stress, when we're so wrapped up in ourselves and our worlds that we need something to help us achieve a sense of remove? Curiously, as Robert Hunter became more enmeshed in golf, he actually became *more* radical. Hunter was very much a product of his time, which is a polite way of saying that there are parts of *Poverty* that scan as shockingly racist to the modern reader. (Don't get him started on the Irish, for example, or skull shapes.) This sort of paternalistic racism was common among reformers of the early 1900s, but that by no means makes it OK, and it's probably one of the reasons that *Poverty* is read by approximately no one today. Which is what makes the tone of his next book, *Socialists at Work* (1908), even more remarkable. He writes that reading W. E. B. Du Bois's *The Souls of Black Folk* was liable to replace a white person's sense of racial superiority with "a humiliating sense of shame" for having once felt superior to others. He rails against capitalism and urges his readers to check out the *Communist Manifesto*. Socialism, he believed, was coming to nations throughout the world "to destroy wage-slavery, and to raise what are now the subject classes into a position of dominant influence."

Yet simultaneously, he and his wife had begun vacationing regularly at Pinehurst, where, even with his kooky politics and relative inexperience with the game, he managed to win multiple club championships and even come in second at Pinehurst's North & South Amateur Championship, considered back then to be one of the "Majors" of amateur golf. I would have imagined that having a full-on Socialist, let alone a famous one, in their midst would have made the titans of industry in Pinehurst uncomfortable, or even outright hostile. Here was a guy who, in addition to beating them on the course, was actively working to break down their own system. This was a time during which political violence, whether it was lone anarchists carrying out assassinations or unions getting into skirmishes with the National Guard, was commonplace, and there was legitimate cause for concern that class tensions might boil over into revolution.

Yet Hunter's status as a "salon socialist" (a name given to him by Teddy Roosevelt) appears to have been seen as a curio by the greater Pinehurst community. Local newspaper archives show that the local library always stocked his books, and when it was announced that he would be running for Senate in Connecticut as the Socialist Party's candidate, one paper quipped that if Hunter was as good a Socialist as he was a golfer, then he'd win the election in a landslide. (Spoiler alert: He didn't.) Maybe it's that the golf course has a leveling influence. It's a place where, regardless of what we believe and who we are in the outside world, we're all trying to navigate the same space, playing by the same rules, on our own, yet side by side. As Hunter later joked in *The Links*, "One inoculated with the virus must swing a golf club or perish."

By the time Hunter got around to writing *The Links*, he'd largely left the Left behind. The one-two punch of World War I and the Bolshevik revolution in Russia kind of killed the Socialist Party in America, because (A) nobody ever really got a handle on whether or not it was more Socialist to be for or against the war, and (B) Lenin's success in taking over Russia suddenly made the possibility of a Socialist party taking control—in America, an ideal to be reached through battling it out at the ballot box—a very real thing that had been achieved through battling it out on the, uh, battlefield. The whole thing made Hunter and his friends squeamish.

The movement began to break into factions, with Hunter championing a more intellectually minded, moderate vision of socialism, leading him to catch heat from both the Left and mainstream society, which was quickly developing a reactionary streak. He couldn't win, so he dropped out. He moved to California to teach at Berkeley, and eventually he teamed up with a designer named Alister MacKenzie, one of the guys he'd consulted for *The Links*, to build Cypress Point, which remains one of the most iconic and acclaimed courses in America today. By the forties, Hunter was nearing the end of his life and had become bitterly suspicious of political extremes on both the right and left. He wrote letters to friends railing against Franklin Roosevelt's New Deal policies and claimed he knew of active Communists working in the U.S. government. He began drafting a memoir (it was never published; however, the Indiana Historical Society provided me with a copy) in which he referred to the Socialist ideal to which he once devoted his life as "a fallacy." He writes of his youthful activism with nostalgic distance, as if his political views were a phase he outgrew, their folly revealed to him with the passage of time.

But today is much more like the early 1900s than it is the 1940s. So many Americans work without benefits, protections, or guaranteed wages, trying to eke out a living on tech platforms that are too new to neatly fit into any existing legal framework. The unprecedented boom in the stock market over the late 2010s and early 2020s, meanwhile, concentrated wealth at the top while the rest of us fought for scraps. And if the precarity faced by millions of Americans wasn't clear before the coronavirus hit, the pandemic brought it all into sharp relief. After being laid off from my job just as America went into COVID lockdown, I went to work as a freelance writer, contributing to publications offering rates that never quite match up to their big names and long-standing legacies. Some days, I submit an $800 invoice for an essay I spent a month working on, and I worry that it will be like this for the rest of my life.

What gives me hope, though, is that more people than ever before are waking up to how screwed they're going to be if nothing changes. Slowly, we're demanding things like universal health care, guaranteed income, protections for gig workers, radical reworkings of the justice system—and people are listening. If nothing else, what once seemed impossible no longer does. The point of working, no matter what they tell you, is not to keep working, to get rich, or to simply survive. It's to stop working as quickly as possible and to do something else. And this, I think, is the ultimate point that Robert Hunter's life gestured toward: The closer we get to full socialism, the more time we'll all have to go off and play golf together.

Chapter Nine

HOW GOLF HELPED ME LEARN TO LET GO

I WILL NEVER forget the day it happened, mainly because it was a thing that does not happen to adults. The thing was this:

I, an adult, was bullied. On a golf course. By other adults.

The circumstances leading up to the bullying were normal enough. I'd had insomnia the night before, so in order to tire myself out enough that it wouldn't happen again, I drove to Duke University, whose golf course is horribly hard but compact enough to walk pretty easily. When I got there, the starter, aka the air traffic controller of the links, had me tee off on the back nine so that I could play the front nine later, which often happens when a course is crowded and you're just a single golfer trying to get in a full round.

My golf game comes and goes; sometimes my shots follow a predictable pattern, and sometimes they go all the hell over the place. Today, I was in a transition period between the two extremes, and I sent my first drive skittering along the left side of the fairway, hoping it'd veer right at the last possible moment in a gentle fade toward the green. This did not happen, and instead my ball ignobly rolled into the woods, dying a tragic death on some mulch. The fairways at Duke are narrow, designed to give even elite collegiate golfers a challenge, so I don't know what else I was expecting, really. I trudged toward my ball, accepting my fate.

But as this happened—the hitting into the woods, the walking, the feeling of resignation, and so on—I was intercepted, hard, by the two grown men who were about to bully me, but who at the moment were zooming past me in a golf cart so they could dramatically cut the wheel and stop me like a pair of mall parking lot cops. "What the fuck, dude," one said with an air of unearned but by no means inauthentic authority. His hat complemented his shirt, which matched his socks, which complemented his belt, which matched his shoes, which complemented his shorts. In other words, he wore the same clothes that everyone has to wear at a golf course, but unlike me, he dressed like he meant it.

"You can't just jump in front of us," his buddy said.

"I . . . didn't?"

One of them, I'm not really sure which, because I had a hard time telling them apart, went, "We got three groups behind us, and yes you did, shit's not cool."

"I mean, I'm sorry if you're upset, but the starter told me to play the back nine first and to go off quick, so I did. If he had me cut y'all, I'm not happy about that, either." I made conciliatory gestures and grabbed my six-iron with the intention of hitting a low punch shot out of the woods so I could get out of their way.

"Just so you know," they said in unison, "we play fast." OK, they didn't say it in unison. Maybe they alternated words. They'd gotten the impression, falsely, that I'd knowingly and wantonly cut them off, and were letting off some steam based on their incomplete picture of the situation. That's lamentable, but at least it's understandable. Hopefully, within a couple of holes they'd have forgotten I even existed.

Cooler heads, sadly, did not prevail. Neither did diplomacy or tact or compromise or anything else of that nature. I began to suspect that the bags of sleeplessness under my eyes were not cause for sympathy to these people, but instead a sign of weakness. As I steadied myself for my next shot, I heard the *thwack* of someone else's golf club hitting someone else's golf ball. One shot sailed over my head, then another, and—wait, were they passing me without asking?

In the interest of, I don't know, saving face maybe, I waved at them and asked, "Y'all wanna play through?" as they drove their golf cart past me. They did not acknowledge my presence, the mythical groups behind them did not materialize, and they proceeded to futz around on each green, chatting and taking extra putts even though there was no one in front of them and I was maybe fifty yards away. To this day, my failure to resist their act of overt aggression makes me want to collapse into a puddle of interpersonal inadequacy.

To be clear, this is probably the rudest thing one can do on a golf course without getting kicked off. False accusations of Golf Crimes are bad, forced play-throughs are worse, and taking extra putts on every single green, thereby forcing the person behind you to wait five minutes on each hole, is just twisting the knife. Two holes into my round, I caught one of them saying, "Honestly, this whole pandemic thing is just as fake as anthrax was after 9/11," to which the other responded, "Yeah, man, at best it's an excuse for people to get out of going to work and stuff." They didn't care about the contradictions inherent in the fact that they were having this conversation at a golf course on a Monday, because this is not how these things work.

A quick story: There were times when my high school golf team was sort of like *The Bad News Bears* without any of the heart-warming stuff. I mentioned this earlier in the book, but once we were playing a practice round and my friend Brett was standing too close to my other friend Derek (not their real names) as he was taking a practice swing with a four-iron; Derek swung back harder than he should have, and on its way up, the club connected directly with Brett's left cheekbone. As we walked Brett back to the clubhouse, propping him up in case he passed out, we could hear Brett's face crunch with each slow, excruciating step. When Derek wasn't crying, he was telling Brett every way he could think of that he wished he could take it back, he was sorry, oh my God holy fuck dude please be OK, you can punch me in the face as hard as you want to I totally deserve it. Brett was a Mormon, though; he wasn't into that. Most of the girls always thought he was the hottest guy in our year, and after the doctors at St. Luke's put a plate in his face and it was all healed up, the consensus didn't change a whit.

There was also this low-level aggression that most of the players carried with them all the time, a glee at the misfortune of others that was, for much of my junior year on the team, directed at me, for being a worse player than them, for having junky hand-me-down clubs, for being clumsy and awkward and always doing homework on the bus back from matches. Mostly, the good players didn't like me because they were good and I was bad, and so they didn't really like talking to me; the next year, when I got a little better and had a car that I'd give them rides to practice in while playing rap music, they decided I was mostly OK, and I decided the feeling was mutual. We'd play together whenever we were all back from college sometimes; one summer, I was on steroids to help heal a fractured finger, and one of them hooked me up with some weed so I could sleep.

People change, but the way they make you feel stays with you, long after you even associate it with them. And that's probably why my interaction with those guys at the Duke golf course is burned into my head: It brought back every feeling of inadequacy, of awkwardness, of trying but so obviously failing to fit in, that I had experienced as a high school golfer.

I wish I could say that the attitude the dudes who bullied and then passed me gave off wasn't representative of golf as a whole, but it kind of is sometimes. It's a sport that draws in both the privileged and those who fantasize about privilege, placing them in an environment designed expressly for their enjoyment. Obviously, this isn't a golf-specific phenomenon, but the game's tendency to incarnate a mentality that "the customer is always right" can make hitting the links as annoying as, say, taking a cruise (but with way fewer germs). Besides, golf tends to attract white men, and white men as a demographic group tend to lean relatively conservative. And once you start talking about people at fancier golf courses, whether they're private or public, the likelihood of their possessing a conservative streak only increases—after all, if you've got the money to be there in the first place, then you've probably got more money than most and, therefore, a vested interest in hanging on to it. A dislike of paying your taxes can lead people into some truly weird political territory.

That's without even mentioning golf courses themselves. During the late 1990s and early 2000s, a wave of golf communities sprang up throughout the nation but especially in the South, ranging from challenging courses surrounded by multimillion-dollar mansions to humble homes amid a sea of pedestrian fairways. When it came to the high-end projects, the developers often wrangled a big-name golf course architect, provided a budget in the millions, and said to play God over a plot of land. The architect would preferably be a superstar auteur such as Pete Dye or Tom Fazio, whose punishing and beautiful designs drew media interest and the potential to host professional tournaments, but an established PGA pro who built courses on the side, like Davis Love III or Ben Crenshaw, would do in a pinch. These guys would move heaven and earth (or, to be less metaphorical, just lots and lots and *lots* of earth) to create lakes, valleys, and hills upon a previously unsculptured plot. They imported geographically improbable grasses, trees, and shrubbery, keeping them alive through mounds of fertilizers and elaborate sprinkler systems. The end results would often be ecstatically beautiful, fantastically difficult, and almost prohibitively expensive to maintain.

More often than not, the developers behind these projects weren't truly in the business of golf courses, but instead the business of real estate: These courses essentially served as marketing materials for the lots being cleared and houses being erected that they hoped to sell to customers. And the communities that they helped market were part of a larger wave of preplanned neighborhoods throughout the nation—the spiritual successor to the suburban boom that had come a generation before. Golf courses were great for these places, hypothetically, because even if a prospective buyer didn't actually play golf, having a fairway in your backyard meant predictability. It wasn't like you risked waking up one day and seeing a bunch of construction equipment putting up something that would block the nice view from your back porch. It was always going to be a golf course, the thinking went—and if you were the type of person who'd prefer to live in one of these places over a bustling downtown or more urbanized neighborhood, I can only assume that stability (or golf) was probably extremely important to you.

Once enough properties had been sold to turn a snazzy profit, the developer would sell the course itself—usually to a company specializing in golf course management, and usually at a steep discount—and then move on to the next spontaneously generated prefab paradise. By the early 2000s, the rate at which golf courses were being built in America had begun to outstrip that of new golfers entering the sport, yielding a 13 percent decrease in the number of potential golfers per course from 1990 to 2000.

That should have probably been a signal that the golf industry was being flooded with a supply of golf that outstripped its demand. The thing about markets is that, as a general rule of economics, they like to achieve equilibrium. In the real world, that would have meant either closing some golf courses or convincing more people to play golf. The first option would have been easier than the second, but only the second would have led to everyone with a golf course making more money. There was a third option, too, I guess, which was to somewhat slow down the pace at which new golf communities were being constructed, hope that the ongoing popularity of Tiger Woods would lead more people to the sport, and assume that the housing market wasn't going to help cause a massive, society-changing recession in a few years. This is the one that, as a whole, the golf industry decided to go with.

My first job was at one of these communities-to-be, a high-end construction in the foothills of the Blue Ridge Mountains that was being overseen by Tom Fazio himself. The year was 2005; I was fifteen; the town closest to the course had a population that was somewhere in the low three figures. I worked on the grounds crew along with ten or so other kids from my high school, tending to the half of the course that had already been built while the other nine holes were still under construction. Or at least, that's what the course's management had in mind for us. We were more concerned with slacking off as much as humanly possible, preferably while joyriding around on an unfathomably valuable piece of industrial equipment. It rained like hell that summer, and we'd pray for days when the downpour would hit just as we got to work in the hope of spending a few hours in the leaky barn where we clocked in, racking up idle hours as everyone (except me) smoked cigarettes and everyone (including me) entered into shit-talking contests that I always lost.

My main memory from that summer is feeling the wind whipping my face as I rode shotgun in an ATV being driven by a guy I'll call Clayton, going forty-five miles per hour down a steep gravel road that connected a cluster of lots to the barn. Clayton sold weed and was the only person I was friends with who'd dropped out of high school; he told me the sole reason he took the job was so his mom wouldn't ask where all his money came from. Lots on the course started at something like $100,000 each, and the only way to become a member was to buy one of them. The course was to be patient zero for an impending golf explosion in the area: Just a few miles away, another group of developers had secured the necessary permits to build another golf destination featuring a course designed by none other than Arnold Palmer. It was the trickle-down wishful economic thinking of George W. Bush's first term at its finest: Rich investors had decided that there was gold in our hills—or at least, that our hills were gold and that people would want to play golf on them. They enticed the locals with the promise of building luxury homes and filling them with a battalion of wealthy tourists, a self-sustaining stream of construction projects and service jobs that would never run dry. In retrospect, though, it felt more like Harold Hill coming to River City in *The Music Man* than anything else.

All the rain that summer threw a monkey wrench in the developers' schedule for completing the remaining nine holes, and it made our job to keep the existing half of the course from going to hell. So much of my summer was spent shoveling dirt onto eroded slopes, tamping down loose turf, re-spreading seeds that had washed away. Probably one day a week we would have to load up the bed of a Polaris ATV with two-foot-wide strips of sod and repair the side of the hill that had been built up so steeply that it disrupted the natural flow of rainwater, sending the sod we'd laid the previous week sliding down into the woods. We'd start by recovering the loose strips of old turf that hadn't started rotting from sitting in the hot and the wet and putting them back in their place the best we could, then laying new strips along the hill, arranging them in a neatly staggered pattern as if they were bricks in a wall. As one of us laid, another would follow with a hammer and a pocket full of lawn staples; behind them, someone followed with a heavy iron tamp to pack everything down. Each week, I hoped this would finally be the time the sod's roots fused with the earth, and each week I found myself yet again taking part in this Sisyphean task.

I honestly can't remember whether we finally got the sod to stick. Seeing as the bit of the hill we'd been working on was the far side of an elevated green and therefore would be looked at by approximately no one ever, I wouldn't be surprised if our bosses just finally gave up. Right around the time they finally finished the course enough to open it up to the public, the bottom dropped out of the housing market, leaving behind a world-class golf course bound by a halo of nearly unsellable lots. A few years later, the course's owners opened the place up to the public in a bid to get someone, anyone, to play golf there. A few years after that, they gave up and shut the course down altogether.

In my early thirties, when I was back home visiting my parents, my partner and I drove out there to check it out; I imagined showing her the spectacle that was a once-resplendent golf course being slowly reclaimed by the forests that had been cleared to create it, maybe taking a pitching wedge and trying to stick a few shots on the cursed and now-overgrown green whose sides I'd long ago spent so much time sodding. A kiosk now stood in the middle of the winding road leading up to the old barn, manned by a chipper college student who informed us that the community—they'd finally managed to build some houses there!—was closed to everyone except homeowners and their guests.

I tried explaining that we just wanted to look at the old golf course because I'd worked there in high school and that we wouldn't bother anybody. But, firmly and steadfastly, with the forced cheer of someone who was in no way being paid enough to have to deal with anything beyond letting familiar people drive their familiar cars past her kiosk, she refused to let us in.

My face went flush. In that moment, I cared about that golf course more than I ever had when I'd worked there. In my own small way, I had helped make it exist, to keep it beautiful, and now that it had gone to hell, I couldn't even survey the damage. Or maybe what I wanted more than anything was a sense of closure, visual confirmation that all the dumb tasks I'd been given in high school had truly been for nothing. Whatever it was that I sought, I was being denied it by the arbitrary whims of an unseen and all-powerful homeowners' association. The ability to say, "I am at a place that is mine and not yours due to various decisions we have both made involving our respective histories of capital accumulation and allocation," is inherently part of what you pay for when you join a private golf course. I guess I'd just never realized that for some people, that's the product they're actually buying.

• • •

One day, my partner and I got an itch that wouldn't stop until we moved to the North. Not like Canada or anything, just somewhere north of North Carolina. We settled on Philadelphia. We'd been visiting and loved it, it was relatively affordable, and they had golf there. We gave ourselves six months to get out of town—enough time to tie up loose ends down in Durham, but still so soon that it felt like every move we made was drawing us inexorably toward the moment of leaving.

I started emailing country clubs in Philly asking about memberships. This was partially because the hardest part of leaving is having to say goodbye. I wanted to get my mind off logistical things like considering the dimensions of all the different U-Haul trucks, reading Amazon reviews of seemingly identical cardboard moving boxes, having to call my parents to ask if this plate or that rickety desk from my childhood was secretly a family heirloom or just some crap they'd gotten when they were younger and later foisted onto me (it was almost always the latter). It broke my heart to help my partner get rid of the plants in our garden, watching as she gave a final sniff to each sprig of rosemary and thyme, thanking them for enriching our lives, before we emptied their pots. Paralyzed by the anxiety of letting go, we failed to see many of our friends before we left, hoping we'd at least told them we were leaving and trying to discern which of them would be insulted if they found out on Instagram that we skipped town.

Reviewing club brochures, triangulating drive times to courses from our new address, making spreadsheets comparing each place's initiation fee plus monthly dues plus dining minimum to try to discern which was *truly* the best value, and listening to friendly membership directors tell me about guest policies and pool privileges and how their facility has a state-of-the-art golf simulator for the winter months helped remind me that weren't just packing our shit in a truck and driving into the abyss. There was something on the other side.

Besides, Philly is a country club town. It doesn't have a ton of public golf courses worth playing, and the ones that are tend to be way too expensive. Even those are often crowded as hell, and seeing as I wanted to keep playing regularly, preferably somewhere that would allow me to knock out a quick nine holes after work, I began acclimating myself to the idea.

Despite its cultural connotations, the term "country club" doesn't really mean anything. It's just a place where, rather than paying for a single round of golf, you pay by the month, quarter, or year for unlimited to access to a course. Their fees can range from fifty bucks a month into the thousands, and the hypothetical country club I imagined myself joining charged near the lower end of the spectrum. When the weather's nice and there's enough daylight, I've typically tried to play golf at least twice a week at a minimum, supplemented by a couple of quick trips to the driving range. After looking at the rates for the public courses near my house, I realized that joining a country club might actually make my debilitating golf habit *cheaper*.

To put it in terms an economist might use, golf as a product is not a "luxury good"—something that, due to its intrinsic value or scarce supply, will always cost a lot. There's so much untouched land in this world, whether we're talking about an abandoned lot in the city, a field in the country, or a stretch of desert off the highway, that a person could easily repurpose into a golf hole with little more than a lawn mower and a shovel (or, in the case of the desert, just a shovel). Similarly, actual golf equipment is in ready supply at basically any thrift store. So the experience of playing golf—the thing you pay for—should not be expensive, because we can always figure out a way to do some golf-like activity for free. Instead, the commodity that is "the golfing experience" is a "status good," which derives its price from the socially constructed myth that golf is a sport of the elite. And though it's a product of magical thinking, that doesn't change the fact that the people who buy into this false assumption and view it as a good thing are often the sorts of people you find at country clubs. It's not even like they're deeply unpleasant people to interact with or anything, just that their enthusiasm about being in the in-group often has an unfortunate side effect of their casually denigrating those on the outside.

When you go play golf alone, the pro shop people tend to pair you with at least one other person in order to maintain the pace of play throughout the course. Sometimes, my playing partners have been minor nightmares: club-throwers and tantrum-tossers, compulsive gamblers, people complaining that the course isn't challenging enough before slicing their tee shot into the woods, dudes with goatees, that sort of thing. And then there are the people who feel way too comfortable letting their casual racism, misogyny, and homophobia slip out just because they think the golf course is their "safe space" or something. It goes without saying that these people are the worst, and if you've ever met an adult who's lightly tormented a waiter, thinking it was funny, then you know exactly the type of person I'm talking about.

I didn't like the idea of being around people who thought like this. Or maybe I didn't like the idea that people might think that *I* thought like this, and that they'd know enough about golf to make a distinction between country club people and non–country club people.

Despite my hesitation and outright self-consciousness about the whole endeavor, I reached out to at least ten country clubs about possibly joining. Some I disqualified immediately: one for tacking on weird fees to their monthly rates (shady!), another telling me I needed to be nominated for membership by at least two of their current members (fratty!), and a couple for not responding to my emails (disappointing!). But one, a smaller place just outside the city, felt perfect. The membership was a mix of suburban retirees and young people living in the city, the price was right, and the membership director and I ended up talking on the phone for forty-five minutes about our lives. I told him I'd rediscovered golf as a way to overcome depression; his path to the game was similar. This was just his day job, he told me—his real passion, he said, was the memoir he'd spent the past five years working on, writing in snatches when he got the chance.

Offhandedly, he mentioned that he used to be a professional dog rescuer, which was a thing that I had not realized was a viable career path.

This is not a country club person, I thought, *and if this place is good enough for him, I bet it's good enough for me*. I told him I loved the idea of joining, but I needed to think about it and get back to him.

It all made sense on paper, but I just couldn't bring myself to pull the trigger. I was judging myself for joining the most benign, me-friendly country club I had found, even though (A) nobody else cared, and (B) I hadn't even signed up yet. But millennials occupying similar political real estate to what I do tend to feel complicit in everything, obsessing over how we're unconsciously contributing to the ills of the world. *How is what I'm buying and saying and doing hurting or helping society, and is there some sort of social equivalent to a carbon tax I can pay to offset the bad stuff I've inadvertently done?* Holding ourselves accountable is good, but there's a difference between that and refusing to give yourself and others a break. Not to be too reductive, but social media has changed the way we interface with the world, turning every action and interaction into an opportunity for performance. In doing this, we let power off the hook, and we even create the space for it to co-opt our good intentions so that they might mask their ill ones.

Often, we accept the grip that the powers that be hold over our lives and come to view them as so totalistic that there's no way they could be toppled or even changed at all, except by millions of individuals doing little good deeds in every direction. But who are we helping by doing this? Are we influencing others to do better, or have we inadvertently created a hermetic, country club–like sphere of our own, this exclusive group modeling good behavior for one another, while the nonmembers go about their business as usual—and, in the case of conservative culture warriors, actively antagonize us?

Because here is the thing: The world is full of rotten systems and institutions; keeping track of all of them, and attempting to stay on the right side of anything, can cause you to lose your mind. We're under no obligation to actively change the game of golf; none of us are Golf Jesus, because that is not a thing that exists. And besides, by being at a golf course, treating everyone there with dignity and respect, listening to your playing partners so that you can understand their perspectives on the world while expecting the same in return from them, you are, in your own small way, making the game better.

There will certainly be times when you will not, in fact, be able to convince some rando you're playing golf with that it's actually bad to say racist, homophobic, or misogynistic stuff, but you might be surprised to discover that it actually can work. After all, they're stuck with you for eighteen holes, so they've got an incentive to play nice with you. I'm by no means saying that this is the right strategy for *everything*—form a union with your fellow employees rather than trying to single-handedly convince your boss to be nicer, punch Nazis when you see them, go start a commune with your friends and experiment with collectively organized, horizontal societies, and so on. But within the context of golf, we each get to determine what the game means to us and act accordingly.

That, more or less, was the conclusion that I came to after about six weeks of agonizing over whether or not to actually join. I'd just spent a lazy Friday playing with a father and son, both named Tim, at a course in New Jersey about an hour away, and while I'd had a great time, the pace of play was slower than drying paint, half the greens were closed off, and we were forced to putt into cups haphazardly jammed into bits of fairway. *Even if the country club sucks, which it probably won't, it'll be better than this*, I thought on the way home. I called the membership director to let him know I wanted in.

He wasn't there, so I shot him a text message, the de facto voice mail for all humans born since the Carter administration.

The membership director never texted back.

I felt an irrational pang of rejection once I realized I probably wasn't going to hear from him. Like everything else in life, golf can be a source of pain as much as it is of joy, especially if you have a deep emotional investment in it that causes you to overanalyze everything. Was I being rejected because I wasn't a country club person at heart? Had they googled me and seen that I'd written multiple articles that had the word "fuck" in the title?? Did they hear about the time I'd bought all those Four Lokos for Steve???

None of those things, I soon realized, had happened. Instead, the guy was probably just busy and forgot to get back to me. He was just a person trying to get by, the same as me. Sometimes, things happen, and we don't have to attach a bunch of meaning to them, and that's OK.

Instead, someone else from the club got back to me, saying they'd love to have us come visit. As my partner and I wandered its halls, nobody gave us dirty looks for puncturing the sanctity of *their* private haven. Instead, they waved. Part of the place's draw for me was its affordability, which is generally incompatible with snobbery—if you want to go somewhere and be a snob, you go somewhere expensive. Instead, it was just a place where people hung out and did their thing. It was warm and welcoming, so much so that it helped me remember that things don't have to be forever loaded with the same meaning. There are times when we can let go of our preconceptions and simply let things be.

In the end, I joined the hell out of that country club. I haven't regretted it a bit.

Chapter Ten

HOW GOLF TAUGHT ME TO APPRECIATE WHAT I HAVE

BEFORE WE MOVED to Philadelphia, we decided to spend most of July and August in Brooklyn, at my partner's parents' place near Prospect Park. They had bought it back when the neighborhood was the third worst in the city, her dad told me. He grew up in Alphabet City, drove a cab to put himself through college, went on to become a podiatrist, and ended up inventing a new type of Velcro shoe. (More accurately, he figured out a system for securing your foot into a shoe with Velcro, and he sold the patent to a major sporting company for a minor sum.) To this day, he's constantly vigilant about alternate-side parking and can eyeball the required fifteen feet from his rubber bumper buddy to the hydrant. He told me all his tricks before they left us to house-sit while they went on a trip. "Never drive into the city, except for dinner, because the meters stop running at seven. And you should really do it only on a Monday or a Thursday night, because when you come back you can grab a Tuesday or a Friday spot close to the house and move it the next day when everyone's at work. If everything's filled up, you can always double-park and do work on your laptop during the street-cleaning hour, or if you can't do that, just double-park and leave a note with your phone number on your windshield so someone can call you and ask you to move your car if they've got to get out. Or just go get your groceries during street cleaning. That's what I do."

Our first night there, I misread the hours on the sign and didn't go to move my car until after the street-cleaning period had ended. Miraculously, I did not receive a ticket. I ended up doing this three more times during our stay, forgetting to move my car a little less unintentionally each time. The last time it happened, mine was the only car left on the Friday side, and I had to race to beat a meter enforcer, ticket machine in hand, to my car and beg to be allowed to move it. The person said sure, whatever.

Most alternate-side parking days, though, I decided to hit the links. It was a fifteen-minute drive to one golf course, a place called Dyker Beach, and thirty to another, Marine Park. They're both owned by the city and equally a rip-off, but Marine Park's a nicer course, so it's always more crowded.

But even an uncrowded golf course in New York City is populated unlike any other on this earth. Here they take the subway and buses to play, lugging clubs for blocks at both ends. They sit in traffic on the BQE, the Belt, the West Side Highway, the FDR Drive, waking up at five thirty for an eight thirty tee time. There are almost no driving ranges here, either, so for beginners it's truly sink or swim and let God sort it out.

Either by design or providence, golf is slow in New York. Look left and it's lush as North Carolina, look right and it's an impossibly packed street with life moving a thousand miles a minute. Or: "It's a fuckin' zoo out here," said Eddie, a man who started talking to me in the Dyker bathroom. He wore a New York Mets polo and a Titleist cap with the Mets logo etched on the side and contorted syllables in ways that I had previously assumed were only theoretically possible. "And the first cut? They gotta do something about that shit. I lost three, four fuckin' balls out there."

"That's the city of New York for you," I said, complaining about the city government as my partner's father had taught me to do. Among true New Yorkers, I have been told, hatred of local bureaucracy is one of the few things uniting the citizens of the most diverse city in the world, a hatred so strong that it is present even among those who work for it.

"Don't even get me started about the bunkers," he continued, taking my light complaint as an invitation for him to keep going. "They were supposed to fix them last summer, but did they? Hell no. You gotta take a drop every time—it's all rocks in there."

He didn't even get to the bees, which I had come to loathe and fear; for some reason, most of the sand traps at Dyker were infested with them: big ones, maybe wasps, buzzing incuriously as you gingerly removed your ball from their territory. I had a feeling that it was these loathsome insects that kept the city from putting new sand in, because whoever had the task would get stung, and either no one wanted to be the one to fall on that particular sword or maybe the city didn't want to fork over the medical bills that would inevitably occur in the event of the stinging. Either way, the city seemed to be engaged in an elaborate game of three-dimensional chess whose outcome had left the bunkers to the wasps.

But the thing is, golf in New York is special. Between the traffic and the slow play guaranteeing that it'll take up your whole day, the search for lost balls in the tall rough, the need to hit out of divots in the fairway, the slow greens, and the fact that you could literally die out there, it's a commitment. So you'd better savor it. And much like living in the city itself, the hope is that you reach a point where endurance sublimates into enjoyment, a pride that by simply being there and going through it, your will has grown strong, strong like a DMX video or the guy I saw uptown doing resistance band exercises on a sign pole—which, now that I think about it, sounds like a thing that would be in a DMX video.

Eddie also hated that the grill was open only on the weekends, by the way. It was apparently open on a Monday the last time he was here, but now they've got a sign up saying it's open only on Saturdays? "What the fuck's up with that? I've had it with this place. Ehhh, I'll be back next Tuesday," he said. "I'll see you then, if you're around."

I didn't see Eddie on Tuesday, because on Tuesday I played at Marine Park, which is a golf course in a park that is also called Marine Park and is at the ass end of Brooklyn. Like a lot of things in the city, it's a physically ancient place in a state of constant rejuvenation. Today, it's the largest park in Brooklyn, and like more than a few parks in the city, it has existed as both a literal and metaphoric trash heap, but it's pretty nice now.

Part of Marine Park had once been an island marsh, donated to the city by a naturalist; but when the villainous urban planner Robert Moses, whose machinations shaped the city in ways both seen and not, got his hands on it, he threw so much trash on the island that it fused with the mainland. When he was building the

Belt Parkway in Brooklyn, he dealt with the sand displaced for the new road by dumping it on the trash in Marine Park, which, if I understand correctly, somehow inadvertently caused the marsh to come back.

When they built the golf course in 1963, the city added in a layer of asphalt for good measure, but the site remained a miasma of filth, lawlessness, and decay that would be impossible to believe except for the fact that it existed. A 1965 *New York Times article* described an army of "teen-agers with bows and arrows hunt[ing] rats" that "run in and out of junked automobiles, rotting mattresses, upholstered chairs and sofas with their stuffing cut open, abandoned baby carriages, wooden doors, bedsprings, refrigerators, tires, beer cans, milk containers and discarded foodstuffs." (This is to say nothing of the fact that today, Marine Park Golf Course is *one of the preferred locations in the city* to illegally release live raccoons captured elsewhere in the city.)

Maybe it's the legacy of the Great Teens versus Trash Rats War of 1965, or maybe it's that in the 1800s, the land was home to a gigantic facility where horses went to die, and that's got to be horrific karma, but for whatever reason, the golf course on its grounds, while beautiful, challenging, and uniquely in tune with what passes for the natural world in New York, is also home to the largest mosquitoes this side of science fiction.

I first saw them on the third tee box, following a long par 4 that traced the highway on one side and the water separating the mainland from Dead Horse Island (technically, now an isthmus) on the other. They looked like flies at first, a minor annoyance, but then I looked down and noticed a splotch of blood on my sock. I then saw a not-a-fly-actually-a-mosquito locked into my other ankle, and I got the disconcerting sensation of knowing that I should have felt pain yet, due to whatever's in mosquito saliva, couldn't feel a thing. Instead, I experienced the anticipation of an itch and smacked it as hard as I could. This caused another splotch, this one bigger—the result of both blood leaking out of the hole left by the bug and the fact that when I hit the little guy, it exploded—to appear on my sock.

My playing partner for the day, Lou, started hitting his own legs. "My wife's gonna think I got in a fight," he said. He was a recently retired third-rail supervisor for the Metropolitan Transportation Authority, and he came to Marine Park from Staten Island almost every day to get out of his wife's hair. He had braces on both knees, but like any good New York golfer, he walked the course to save the twenty bucks on a cart rental—a stupidly high price on the face of it, I felt, which became even more ridiculous once the first cart they give me started spitting black smoke out the back and I had to get a new one. The good cart had a seat so spongy and deep that I needed to crane my neck to see over the steering wheel. "When you play in the city, you gotta always, always come to Marine Park," Lou said. "Never go out to Dyker. It's a dump."

Lou was a little on the short side and, despite his age, was objectively jacked, and he had the cool jacked-dude thing where it seemed like he'd willed himself to be completely bald so that people got to see the muscles on his skull move around as he spoke. "I got married at nineteen, had a fuckin' kid at twenty, had no idea what we were doing, but you know what? We made it work. I hated my job, I got no cartilage in my left knee, no ACL in my right, both from walkin' on fuckin' subway rocks all day.

But it bought me my house on Staten Island. And now I get to come out here. I love it."

Here was a man who'd spent his life accumulating wisdom, and, now that he was retired, he had all the time in the world to share it. "Hey, listen," he said as he scratched at his bites. "Life doesn't always give you golden fuckin' eggs. But you can still be happy."

To be fair, Marine Park was worth the annoyance of the mosquitoes. It's probably—scratch that, definitely—the best municipal course in the city. (Bethpage, home to the legendary Black Course, is outside the city on Long Island, and the Trump Organization runs a municipal course up in the Bronx, but *until the city's contract with the company is officially severed*, the greens fees are way too high to justify playing there, and that's putting aside any weird moral issues that one may have about playing at the place.) Marine Park was an early design from the important golf architect Robert Trent Jones, and it's about as close to links-style golf as you could hope for on this side of the Atlantic. Its challenges aren't obvious at first. Most of the holes are about the same length and shape, and if you slice off the tee, you'll probably end up on the next fairway. But there are mounds everywhere, both in the fairways themselves and on their borders, full of thick, stringy grass that spontaneously develops claws whenever a ball comes its way. If you find yours, there's no guarantee that you'll be able to hit it out. And the wind!

So much of modern golf, in America at least, is predicated upon the idea of "knowing your yardages." As in, how far do you hit each club? The idea is to dial in your distances, understand which way your ball flies when you misstrike it; on every shot, you take the club that goes the number you need and aim a bit in the opposite direction of your potential miss. For skilled players, regular point-and-shoot golf can become rote, not all that different from, say, archery. On a links course like Marine Park, the wind blows in little swirls that cause balls to wobble through the air, unsteady, until one eddy wins out and you end up wherever they take you. At times, I kept the ball in the back of my stance, leaned on my front foot while sliding the other away from me, and tried to hit a low hook that would roll to its intended destination, but that didn't work either, because Marine Park's fairways are as bumpy as a cobblestone street, and every little curve of the earth presents another variable that simply cannot be accounted for. Even the mosquitoes started to feel like one of the challenges Marine Park threw at me, testing my focus and even my will. I left my bug spray in the car; Lou didn't have any, either. My socks were polka-dotted by the time we were through.

But this is why Marine Park is great. Between the license to complain during the ordeal and the sense of sheer survival you feel afterward, sometimes it's fun to pay money to feel like shit.

• • •

I made it out to Marine Park one more time for an uneventful eighteen before something happened. Due to an unexpected emergency, my partner's parents declared their trip over a month prematurely, and as a result, we had to vacate their place.

We were distraught. We had no plan B; the idea was always to go to Brooklyn in July and hang out until September. I guess it wasn't much of a plan A for that matter, either, but it seemed like the sort of thing that wouldn't come with a lot of contingencies. No matter what, it was over, and if I'd asked any of the New Yorkers I'd been playing with what had happened, they doubtlessly would have said that, somehow, this was Mayor Bill de Blasio's fault.

We had two days, maybe three, to figure out a new plan. We sent texts, made inquiries, asked friends to ask friends, but we did not want to leave yet because we had hoped for one more month there, and there was so much New York left to see. Her parents offered to trade places with us so that we could go upstate, fleeing the city for the Hudson Valley like real New Yorkers. Maybe we could find an Airbnb or a sublet in the city, even though oh my God don't get me started on the prices. Maybe we'd just give up and go home. But no, not the last one. We had one more month of doing left, and, like Parisians in August, we wanted to not be doing it in the usual place.

I called my friend Steve to tell him what had happened. He and his partner were at a wedding in Montana and wouldn't be back until next Monday. Would we want to stay at their place in Philly? We were friends with their roommates, it was an hour and a half away, and we weren't sure what the internet situation was like at the place upstate, so yes. It wasn't golden fuckin' eggs, but it did the trick.

The drive, out of South Brooklyn, down the BQE to the Belt, took us past Dyker, down to where the highway splits—and if you take it left, you get to Marine Park, the memory of which still causes my skin to itch wistfully. We turned onto the Verrazzano Bridge, hit the expressway across Staten Island, and landed on the New Jersey Turnpike.

The transition, from the city to the smokestacks just inside New Jersey whose bleak, blightful smog, we joked, somehow kept New York City running, to the parts of the state that seemingly exist only to provide space for the roads to the Philly suburbs and then into Philly proper, was jarring. The ninety-minute drive was barely long enough to process it all, or anything for that matter.

Two days later, I picked up my friend Allie at her place in the Fishtown section of the city. We went to an "executive course" to the northwest. Why they call them that I have no idea. Just one of those things, I guess, or maybe executives are so busy that they can't play eighteen full holes unless they're all par 3s and 4s.

Allie hadn't played golf since she was in high school, but she was from Florida. "Golf's sort of genetic there," she joked. She learned how to play from this dude who operated a driving range in the parking lot of an abandoned Walmart, she said. Or it was something like that, one of those sorts of things that people from Florida say all matter-of-fact even though it's the weirdest thing you'll end up hearing all week.

It turned out that Allie was pretty good at golf. She hit the ball straight, which is the hardest part, and immediately figured out how to run the ball on the green. It was ninety-seven degrees out, and we drank Miller Lights from the pro shop, whose main utility seemed to be to provide us with more liquid to sweat out. Her wife was out of town, she said, and she was glad I was here because she was getting bored out of her skull. After nine holes, we ducked into the pro shop and I helped her pick out some used clubs, so next time she didn't have to rent any. Driver, five-iron, pitching wedge, and putter.

"Don't you wanna get, like, some other stuff?" I asked.

"Nah, I should get good with these first," she said. There's something to that: Most people carry more golf clubs than they actually use. They also have a tendency to lean on the clubs they really like, inventing new ways to hit different shots with them, to the point that they kinda-sorta render other clubs in the bag superfluous. Allie knew that intuitively.

• • •

Then life handed us more lemons. One of Steve's roommates was suddenly feeling sick and had just hung out with someone who had just tested positive for COVID. Which meant that they probably had COVID, too. I found out as I was out getting iced coffee, and by the time I opened the door to the living room, everyone was wearing a mask.

And so we fled to Emilie's parents' empty Airbnb in upstate New York. Displacement felt bad, but at least we were used to it. We weren't sure whether or not the internet worked well enough to do video calls or if it even worked at all, but, hey, what the hell.

The drive up was frantic, anxious. I nearly swerved into a truck in Jersey, and up on the Taconic Parkway, the tire pressure monitor in my car suddenly announced that all four tires were dangerously low, causing me to pull onto the shoulder and get out to check them with my eyes. But I forgot to put the car in park, leaving it to lurch forward a few feet while traffic whooshed past; I jumped back in the driver's seat like I was Vin Diesel and slammed on the brakes. The whole thing nearly gave us both heart attacks—but on the bright side, the tires were fine.

We made it up to Columbia County, where we were greeted by a gravel road that led to the gravel road that led to another gravel road where the Airbnb was. It was so dark that I missed two turns in a quarter-mile span, first driving past the initial gravel road and then accidentally pulling into the wrong driveway, stopping only after we found a sign reading NO AIRBNB THIS WAY. TRESPASSERS WILL BE PROSECUTED.

The place was lovely. It was tucked into the armpit of a hill, new and rectangular and with a tin roof and everything you'd ever need. There was a path from the front door down to a little pond, and perhaps not unrelatedly, we were swarmed by bugs as soon as we stepped out of the car, gnats that followed us toward the inside of the house, which to them must have seemed like an entire universe of light. They weren't Dyker Beach wasps or Marine Park mosquitoes, just bug-bugs, and we were so exhausted and beaten down by the day that we didn't even bother trying to shoo them out.

When people in New York talk about "going upstate," they could mean anything really. But the version of upstate that is the Hudson Valley area is kind of like the European countryside. Everybody's home is within a few minutes of at least one, but usually multiple, little villages, and your world stretches twenty miles in every direction from where you stay. Our villages were Chatham, Old Chatham, Valatie, East Chatham, North Chatham, and Kinderhook, which was the home of Martin Van Buren, the former president whose nickname "Old Kinderhook" apparently inspired the term "OK." When we stretched the bounds of our little existence, we drove out to more metropolitan constellations in western Massachusetts, or Kingston or Hudson. Maybe those names don't mean anything to you, but each has its own character and customs and granular varieties of annoying rich people.

There was a golf course near us that Emilie's dad had previously told me about as we were "making the rounds," as he put it to describe his own peregrinations in Brooklyn saying hi to the other people on their side of the street who'd lived alongside them for decades. ("We never say hi to the people on the other side," he once said. "Whole different neighborhood over there.") The golf course, though, he'd driven past when he was staying in the place, and he thought I might like it, so I checked it out. I ended up going there at least twice a week until we left. It was cheap and never crowded, and I was always the youngest person there besides the pro shop attendant's elementary school–aged son, who every day patiently waited out his summer vacation by playing Nintendo Switch games in the foyer leading to the mazelike locker rooms.

There were gnats there, too, so, so, so many of them, and I got so used to them that I stopped flinching when I accidentally inhaled one. The course was special in the way that many cheap public golf courses are special: Whoever designed it had to work within constraints set by budget or the size of the parcel of land or whatever else, and so they had to get creative in order to keep things interesting. Some of the par 4s would be short enough to reach with your driver, so they made the fairway turn at a ninety-degree angle just to keep people honest; one of the par 5s has two of these elbow-like turns. Then you had a freakishly long par 4 that should have actually been a par 5—another public course staple—as well as what may have legitimately been one of the hardest holes I've ever played. It was a long par 3, uphill over a pond with low-hanging trees on the left, a dogleg cutting to the right, and a thin, elevated green waiting at the end. The trick to getting on the green was to hit a sky-high shot exactly 226 yards with a bit of a fade on it so that it hugged the dogleg and landed soft enough to hold the putting surface. I donated at least half a dozen balls to the forest trying to make this happen, never quite able to make any of my shots cut how I wanted them to. That hole also had the most gnats on it, because of the pond. Only once did I make bogey on it, and I felt like a million bucks afterward.

The farthest I ventured out was to a course sixty miles away, which Golf.com had recently named one of America's top public courses for less than $150. It was a Friday morning when I booked a Monday tee time there; a couple of hours after I gave them my credit card info, a mild hurricane hit the area and I got a call back from them that I'd been rescheduled for Wednesday. When I showed up, the guy in the pro shop informed me that, thanks to all the rain they'd been getting, the place was walking-only that day.

"Can I get a push-cart?" I asked. "My back's killing me. I don't know if I can carry a bag for a whole round."

"Fresh out," he told me. There were carts for sale if I wanted to buy one, though. "Three hundred," he said.

"My back's not hurting that bad," I responded. I shed some weight in my golf bag by dropping off my eight-iron, six-iron, and a hybrid into the trunk of my car and started hoofing it.

Walking a course that was pretty clearly designed to be driven in a golf cart is a singular experience, usually reserved for pro golfers who have caddies or high school and college golf teams who have the zest of youth powering their legs. The paths between holes there forked off in weird directions, and the hole numbers weren't clearly marked; on more than one occasion, I hit a drive in the opposite direction that I should have. But I felt connected to the course in ways that I couldn't have otherwise. My irons and wedges knew what I wanted from them without my having to even ask. Walking in the humid heat had me so tired that I had to sit behind a shed on the sixteenth hole to recover enough strength to finish the round, but it also kept my driver swing smooth, leaving me confident in every shot. I had water, I had energy bars, I had exactly seven golf balls to my name, and sitting there, barely able to think, I fully understood what Lou had meant: Life doesn't always give you golden fuckin' eggs, but even so, a regular egg is special when you look at it the right way.

• • •

Golf's very nature allows for a sense of unhurried appreciation. Simply put, a round of golf is long. There's no way you're getting through eighteen holes in less than three hours minimum, and it's usually more like four or five. You're just out there, taking it all in. When the landscape affects your score, you're incentivized to notice stuff. The more present you are, the more information you have when charting your path to the pin. Play the same course long enough and it unlocks itself, and you form a relationship with each tree, bush, and bump in the earth. Some are your friends, like the little dip in the left side of the fairway that can give your drive an extra fifteen yards of roll, while others, such as a big oak whose branches hang over what otherwise would be an easy and uncomplicated shot at the green, you have to acknowledge and respect—otherwise they'll beat you up.

Being in this zone fosters a sense of wonder. We live on a beautiful earth. Sometimes, I forget that. But then when I'm on the golf course, sometimes I just have to take a step back and say, "Holy cow." Almost anywhere you go, too, there are golf courses, each with its own unique layout, challenges, and clubhouse characters. And yet no matter where you are, the rhythms remain the same—it's only the notes that change. This, to me, makes every golf course feel like home.

Chapter Eleven

HOW GOLF GAVE ME THE STRENGTH TO SUCK

BEFORE I STARTED writing this book, I had about a 15 handicap. I played three times a week, often more. When it was too hot, I went to the driving range, where I could hit balls at my own pace while chugging gallons of water. When it was too cold, I just stayed inside. Golf was just a hobby, something I had only written about a handful of times. It was *my* thing, and there was no pressure to treat it as anything else. I could suck, or I could be great, and no one would know either way.

I began to worry, though, that if I was writing a book about golf, then *I needed to become a good golfer*. On one level, this makes about as much sense as saying that I needed to be able to keep up with UNC–Chapel Hill's basketball team during practice so that I could crank out a history of the program. I mean, in the event that you, the reader, were ever to play golf with me, would it really matter that much if I knocked a few tee shots into a creek? This is a book about how the game of golf can change your life, not one about improving your golf game. And yet, I began having anxiety dreams about not being good enough, that one day I'd open my eyes only to discover that I was being interviewed on the Golf Channel and asked to hit a two-iron over an endless lake, while naked except for a golf glove. The solution, I decided, wasn't to tell my therapist about this stuff or try to translate the ease I felt while on the course into the process of writing this book (or even to make a mental note to pack extra clothes if, by some act of God, I were ever booked to appear on the Golf Channel)—it was to get really good at golf.

I read books on the game, by professional golfers and enthusiastic literary amateurs alike. As I drifted off to sleep at night, I began counting yardages I could confidently hit my clubs: *80 yards and in for my sand wedge, then up to 110 for my gap wedge, 125 for my pitching wedge, 135 for nine-iron, 145 for eight-iron, 155 for seven-iron, 170 for six-iron, 180 for five-iron, 210 for my hybrid, 235 for three-wood, then up to 270 for my driver. Wait oh shit oh fuck oh no goddamn it should I be hitting them farther or am I lying to myself and I can't actually hit them that far? Wait, how does the cold weather change my yardages? Oh God I'll never figure this shit out! How can I write a book if I don't even know how far I can hit a seven-iron????* You know, totally super stuff.

Deep down, I think, I was worried that if I couldn't play brilliantly on demand, or at least possess some level of expertise, then I wouldn't be remotely qualified to evangelize on behalf of the game, as though the validity of what I wrote was directly tied to my ability to shoot even par. Never mind that the entire point of this book is that it doesn't matter whether or not you're good at golf, because the greatness of the game comes from the experience of playing it, not the outcome. I felt like I had to hold myself to a higher—or maybe just different—standard than what I was asking you, the reader, to hold yourself.

This isn't just a me thing. We all have had countless conversations with friends and loved ones assuring them that if they take a step back from the situation and evaluate it objectively, they will realize that whatever they're worried about is not actually that big a deal. But when we try to tell the same things to ourselves, it can be as hard as it would be to actually hit a two-iron over a lake, naked on live TV. This simple truth, that even experts have trouble applying their expertise to themselves, has helped inspire TV shows about brooding detectives, doctors, mobsters, and spies since time immemorial, as well as the old adage that if there are two barbers in town, you should go to the one with the worse haircut, because the barber with the nicer hair probably had his cut by that guy. I know this, and I know that I know this, because I wrote it down on a piece of paper yesterday, and I'm typing it today.

And yet, the more I wrote and read and talked and thought and dreamed about golf, the less I actually understood how to play it. To quote Dostoyevsky's narrator in *Notes from Underground*, "The more conscious I was of goodness and all that was 'sublime and beautiful,' the more deeply I sank into my mire and the more ready I was to sink in it altogether." When your face is an inch away from a big spike that's hanging in the middle of the air, secured by nothing more than your own insistence that there *must* be a spike in your face, you never think to take a step back and see what it is you're actually dealing with.

The spike was my deteriorating golf game, and for months, I just sat there staring at it, wondering what it could have been attached to. Was it the jaw of a T. rex that was very slowly about to eat me? The end of a lance wielded by a pissed-off Renaissance Faire reenactor? Maybe it was part of a new, land-dwelling species of octopus whose tentacles had been hardened into battle-ready instruments. It never occurred to me to get some perspective on the spike, though. Instead, I just sat there, staring and occasionally gesturing at it, hoping it would go away, as instead it grew bigger with every skulled six-iron, duffed three-wood, and chunked chip. I'd managed to learn enough about the game, become so aware of the movements of my body, that I could pretty much tell what I was doing right with my swing, where it was going wrong, and how I was supposed to change it up. But all the knowledge in the world, even when imparted by my teacher Jimmy, couldn't help me execute.

• • •

Most rounds, good or bad, adhered to the same basic narrative arc. They say you're supposed to warm up before you play, preferably by hitting a bucket of balls on the driving range, or at the very least messing around on the putting area so you can get a feel for how fast the greens will roll and a handle over your stroke. But warming up never worked for me; it just made me notice that certain elements of my game hadn't shown up that day. This in turn made me self-conscious, and I'd devise an on-the-fly course management strategy that would keep me from ever having to hit, say, a short iron into a green or a fairway wood off the tee, causing me to feel intense pressure to nail every shot with my driver and seven-iron. And so I would proceed to screw up with those clubs, too. By the fourth hole, I'd have developed a real understanding of which clubs I could rely on that day and which I might as well throw in a wood chipper. Sometimes, I'd hit my driver and all my fairway woods great, duff my irons, chip fine, and spew mediocrity all over the putting green. Or maybe I'd be hooking every single iron and wood but mysteriously chip and putt with an assassin's precision. I was never simply average, always failing in some areas and compensating in others, almost always netting a little less than a bogey per hole.

Once the baseline was established, I would begin to think. I'd realize I had left out at least one pretty major part of a technically correct golf swing, maybe two or three. Like that I wasn't squaring the club's face at impact. Or that I was letting my right elbow drift skyward and keeping it there, rather than tucking it close to my body, forcing my arms to do too much work, robbing me of distance and causing me to impart wild sidespin on the ball. Or that I was off-balance, or swinging too hard, or standing on my heels, or focusing so hard on getting everything right that I was holding my club by the wrong end.

With my mind on so many potential culprits, I would start to lose focus on the actual round itself. It can take several holes for the right clues to trickle out, because like a detective in a bad psychological thriller, the criminal you're investigating . . . is yourself. By the time I figured out the actual issues, I'd usually manage to string a couple of pars together, maybe even a birdie, before the wheels fell off yet again in new and exciting ways. I'd repeat this twice or four times, depending on whether I was playing nine or eighteen holes, and usually ended up with a score of about 87.

Even a bad golf swing can produce a good golf shot, because the main point of swinging a club at all is to strike the ball with the center of the clubface, and to do so in the direction in which you're aiming. This is a difficult thing to do, but it's not *impossible*. Even if there are serious flaws in your swing, if you get lucky the stars will align and your mistakes will complement or maybe offset one another to produce a great-looking golf shot, maybe even a few in a row.

The point of a "good" golf swing then, is to create a repeatable sequence of movements that yield as square a clubface as possible, swung with as much power as possible, with no extraneous motions. After getting this down, then a golfer can start to "shape" the ball: intentionally make it spin a bit in one direction or another in a shot that, when sent right by a right-handed golfer, is called a fade, and when sent left, is called a draw. For example, when Tiger Woods entered his mid-forties, he began to rely upon a gentle fade off the tee, because he found it reliable and easier on his back than trying to kill the ball a billion yards. When perfected, draws and fades are invaluable, because they reduce the variance of a misstruck shot. If I screw up while trying to hit a shot straight and down the center, my ball might spin out to the left or the right, but if I were able to put a Tiger-style fade on it, I'd know it's going to go right—it's just a matter of how far.

For the longest time, I was in a zone where my best shots went slightly right, and my worst ones were screaming slices. But even my "good" shots were objectively bad, because I produced them by having my hands too far out in front of my clubhead while cutting from outside to inside on the ball, creating a glancing blow that robbed me of distance. I used to swing wholly with my arms, which—according to my golf coach Jimmy (as well as the number of balls I lost)—was bad, so I began swinging more with my upper torso. In this period of readjustment, though, I still used my arms too much, causing my elbow to stick out at the top of my backswing like a chicken wing. This led to my needing to readjust my balance on the fly while also turning my body back toward the ball, causing a few good draws and many dive-bombing bad duck hooks. While playing, I'd try to to diagnose my golf problems rather than focusing on what a lovely day it was outside or that I should, despite whatever numbers happened to be on my scorecard, be overjoyed that I was playing golf at all. I could have been anywhere in the world, and I was stuck inside my own head.

It's an overused cliché that the definition of madness is doing the same thing over and over again, expecting a different result. It's also often untrue, and one exception can be found most starkly in golf itself. As in: I would do the same thing over and over again, and the result was *always* different. Meanwhile, hitting one shot perfectly and trying to repeat it was enough to make me go insane. Whenever I brought my clubhead back, there was a maddeningly nonzero chance that I'd come down with it too early, instinctively trying to correct my swing path by pulling the club up with my shoulders. This might lead to the very bottom of my club striking the upper hemisphere of the ball, resulting in a low-flying topped shot (imprecise, bad), or my nearly missing the thing altogether and piddling it forward like four feet (embarrassing, really bad).

All my rounds of golf were bad rounds of golf. That's by golf's metrics, not mine, but on bad days, they became my metrics, too. I let golf tell me that I sucked at it, that I'd never be good, that I'd never find satisfaction even in normalcy.

Then, over the winter of 2021, something magical happened: It rained for two weeks straight. In terms of my own personal comfort and convenience, this was horrible, because winter rain is my least favorite form of weather. Each drop stings like a BB on your bare skin. Puddles develop ice crystals overnight and become viscous pools of solid treachery. I have no way of proving this last one, but I am convinced that this specific type of rain also gave my dog two ear infections, which both she and I really hated. During this time, I couldn't play golf. I could only reflect upon my badness. In one moment, I would yearn to get back on the horse, only in the next to think about all the time the horse must have spent thinking up fun new ways to throw me off again.

But as I stewed and fretted, fretted and stewed, I realized something that the spike and the rain and the pulls and the draws had all but erased from my mind: *Golf is supposed to be fun*. Fun is a part of the human condition. Golf sprang from our impulse to convert boredom into fun. So maybe I just needed to swing in whatever way felt natural for me that day, deal with the consequences as they came, and just give myself over to the game. I'd been trying to force so much on myself, so often and in such volume, that I'd forgotten to actually enjoy golfing. And if I wasn't careful, the thing that had brought me back from a breakdown was going to put me on the brink of another.

When the rain finally subsided, I hadn't played golf in so long that I no longer cared about being good; I just wanted to get back out there. Golf is addicting like that. Its rhythms—the windup and release of the swing, followed by the immediate feedback of watching the shot itself, the flow of tee shot to approach shot to chip to putt, the rattle of the ball in the cup, even the feeling of slinging the bag over your shoulder after you pack up your tools and prepare to do it all over again—form a dance whose steps become so natural that their sudden absence can cause genuine bodily distress. It was like I had an itch inside me, a nagging sensation that I'd forgotten a part of myself somewhere. The notion of finding it while haphazardly spraying balls all over a golf course began to seem deeply appealing.

As I played my first nine holes upon a still-soggy course, fun was what I had. Rather than getting hung up on how I was bringing the golf club back or at which point my legs were bending and stiffening, I just felt grateful that I was where I wanted to be. Everything else began to flow from that simple realization. I let my left thumb snuggle up into my right palm as I gripped the club, because that's what that thumb wanted to do. I even began to close my eyes as I putted in order to just feel my stroke, allowing the fact that I was actually hitting a golf ball to be entirely coincidental. The more I didn't think, the better it felt, and the better I scored as a result. It wasn't that I didn't still hook a shot into the woods or chunk a chip, it was that I no longer gave a damn about those things, and through the power of positive not-thinking, they began to happen less.

After a few rounds employing my new philosophy, a friend and I took a journey to Tobacco Road, a course about an hour from my old house in Durham with a reputation for being more punishing than the Old Testament God. It was designed by a guy named Mike Strantz, a course architect who was almost postmodern in his approach. Because they are products of humans shaping the earth, no golf course is every truly "real," and Strantz's creations did everything they possibly could to remind you that you were not on the coast of Scotland, where you just so happened to be swinging a golf club in a well-manicured field, but that you were, in fact, on a golf course. Tobacco Road contains holes where if you miss the fairway by an inch, your ball will land in a forty-foot-deep bunker that stretches from tee box to green. Others take the idea of risk versus reward to the extreme, offering shortcuts to the green that, if you are even slightly imprecise, will end with your carding an eight. On one, you're asked to hit your first shot onto a fairway that you can't see from the tee box, then land your next shot onto a green that you can't see from the fairway. It is an extremely popular golf course, probably for the same reason that some people are into BDSM: On some level, people like a little pain because it reminds them what pleasure feels like.

In golf, every score tells a story, and every story plays out a bit differently. Even though most courses claim that you should finish their eighteen holes in exactly seventy-two strokes, when it comes to the vast majority of golfers, including plenty of good ones, even coming within spitting distance of shooting par is tantamount to splitting the atom. A more realistic goal is getting around in ninety strokes—otherwise known as bogey golf—but at Tobacco Road, each stroke below that requires an exponentially increasing level of skill, luck, or both. This is a long-winded way of saying that I ended up shooting an 87 at Tobacco Road on that day, and it made me feel like Jack Nicklaus.

For most "good" golfers, an 87 is disappointing. But for an average one, it's an incredible feat. I ended the front nine at Tobacco Road with a 45. I got a par on the first hole, spent far too much of the second hole stuck in a sand trap that Strantz had decided to carve into a hill placed halfway into the fairway, missed far too many makeable par and bogey putts, and had to settle for worse than what I could have earned.

But not giving a shit also meant that I was able to keep up the faith whenever it hit the fan, to push through it with an earth mover so that I could persevere and make it to the completely shitless other side. On the ninth hole, I flubbed a tee shot so poorly that I didn't even make it to the sadistically placed sand trap set at the closest part of the fairway. Eyeing my ball upon the scraggly grass, I counted my blessings: I may have hit my three-wood only the distance I usually send my nine-iron, but I was not in yet another goddamn sand trap.

My options were to (A) attempt to hit a short shot to where my first shot was supposed to be, leaving me with a long approach over more sand traps carved into more hills, or (B) say "screw it" and try to circumvent the entire fairway/hill situation by hitting as long and as high a shot as I could, directly toward the green. My five-wood is my favorite club in my bag, and I had used it multiple times already during the round to hit the exact shot I needed. Fortune favors the bold, and so does Tobacco Road, so I went with option B. No second-guessing, just a quick practice swing to gauge how the uneven ground felt beneath my feet as I tried to make my club move at the speed of a Randy Johnson fastball, and then liftoff.

The ball took off with a dulled *ping!* and wavered for a moment in midair as it reached cruising altitude, as if it were wondering why I thought I could pull this off, before deciding to stick to my plan and plopping onto the top of the hill and settling in a couple of feet away from the green. A chip and two putts later, I earned the greatest bogey of my life.

I started out the back nine with a ho-hum bogey, which I followed up with a birdie on a par 5, thanks to a high-flying four-iron that smacked the slanted back of the green and rolled to within ten feet of the pin. Great. Awesome. Mojo located. Hell yeah. Golf. On the next hole, I celebrated my good fortune by immediately forgetting how to play golf and getting a triple bogey.

When I hit a crappy shot, I get gun-shy about whichever club I hit said crappy shot with, because I now know what I'm capable of when it's in my hands. But seeing as I'd just notched a 7 through hitting bad shots with the aid of a whole third of my bag, I had become a maverick with nothing to lose. Besides, worrying about stuff like that is for people who didn't just miss out on a bunch of golf because of the rain.

The next hole was a long, uphill par 5 with three distinct sections: First, a gulch led up to a fairway where the first shot was meant to land, which then immediately turned right and asked players to carry their second shot over sand traps while not hitting so far that they'd land in yet another and finally one more left turn leading up to a green that was carved within a hill, resembling a dormant volcano. Hit the approach shot too short, and you're in more sand. Too long, and you'll hit a highway. I managed to thread each needle and sink the birdie putt.

I ended the back nine with a 42, which included two birdies, the triple, and a par on the final hole, where I nearly holed out a 65-yard approach shot. Somehow, I managed to shoot my worst ever front nine at Tobacco Road, then my best back nine I'd ever had there, and it added up to the lowest score I'd ever shot on that course. A round of golf will always contain highs and lows, miracles and crushing defeats, and the trick, always, is to maintain an even keel, to tell yourself that you are defined by none of it. You simply are, and that is enough. This, I learned, is the true secret to golf. Hell, and probably to life, too.

• • •

Being kind of bad at golf doesn't mean you care about it less than a scratch player. The magnitude of joy I get from the game, and that you can get, too, does not increase or diminish based on the number written upon a scorecard. What's more, being a mediocre golfer may very well offer *more* opportunities to find joy within the game, because there is so much more to learn, discover, and experience. The chip that helps me save double bogey is more important than the four shots that came before it. The drive that flew straight isn't less satisfying because my playing partner blew theirs 50 yards past mine—in fact, they're not even related, because, outside a tournament, golf, regardless of what people tell you, isn't a competition. It's its own thing.

The long, side-hill putt whose lagging path to the hole requires me to aim forty-five degrees right of the hole can write a ticket to my own personal thriller in three acts as it works its way up the incline, losing speed as it curls before hitting a slope and accelerating yet again, compelled by gravity as it builds to a climax, rolling, do or die, toward the pin. As the adrenaline shoots through my hands and chest and veins and all the other bits and bobs of my body, and I try to harness this jumpy energy into superhumanly willing the ball to drop into the cup, bracing for its fall—and even when I miss by an inch and it rolls four feet past—I feel proud that, even if only for a moment, perfection was within reach.

CONCLUSION

I BEGAN THIS book with a quote from Jack Nicklaus's book *Golf My Way*: "If there's one thing golf demands above all else, it's honesty." It's worth repeating here, I think, because this, ultimately, is the most important lesson that I have taken from golf. It's not like I was a compulsive liar who picked up a golf club and magically turned into someone who told the truth no matter what, but playing such a frustrating and rewarding game has helped me become more honest with myself about my emotions, insecurities, fears, outlook, priorities, desires, and values.

In other words, golf has helped me recognize and accept myself. When people ask me why I play, I tend to overshare. I will tell them that I was once so depressed that I couldn't get out of bed, that I moved back in with my parents and could barely take care of myself, and that when I needed something to help rend me from my own moping interiority and place me back into the realm of the physical, I rediscovered this silly and wonderful and life-affirming game. I'm not embarrassed by any of this—it's often our lowest moments, and how we react to them, overcome them, learn from them, that come to define our lives.

It's also worth noting that I don't think that golf is the only way to get here. There's a ton of stuff, from yoga to macrame to splitting wood to reading the collected works of Marcel Proust, that has helped people in similarly dire situations. There's just something about picking a thing and doing it over and over again until it forms the foundation of a practice that really does make people feel good. (And if you are in genuine distress, nothing in the world can replace the work of a mental health specialist and a caring support network. Part of golf is learning to ask for help from the experts, after all.)

What I like about golf, though, is that there are so many different ways to measure whether or not you're getting better. To a certain degree, people believe that "better" is tied to one's ability to lower one's scores, but the more I've played, the more I have learned what a completely arbitrary measure that is. Better might mean learning to use different techniques when you're hitting your shots, or it might mean making more putts, or hitting your shots farther and straighter. It could mean not having to take mulligans. It could mean taking fewer penalty strokes.

To me, getting better at golf means learning. Learning more about what makes the golf swing function, the outcomes that certain clubs are engineered to create, the unique things that our unique bodies prefer to do when swinging each golf club and setting up shots in ways that anticipate those outcomes. Hell, learning more about the actual golf course you're playing on will make you better, because if you understand that a tree has been placed on a hole to offer you something to aim toward, or that a certain part of the green looks flat but in fact is an optical illusion meant to trick you into leaving your shot short, then you have information that can help inform your decisions. Even just learning about golf itself can make you better, because if you find something within its history or culture or any bit of ephemera at all that resonates with you, then you will love it that much more and have that much better a time the next time you hit the links.

Being a golfer is a state of mind. It stays with you even when you're not playing, and if you truly love the game, its absence only makes the heart grow fonder.

In many ways, I am more of a golfer than I was before I started this book. I've taken lessons. I've read deeply about golf's history as well as books on the game in general. (If you're looking for a book of instructions with a literarily jaunty tone, I'd recommend Ben Hogan's *Five Lessons*; for something at the more analytical end of the spectrum, try *The Passion of Tiger Woods* by the anthropologist Orin Starn, whom I'm lucky enough to have shared a few rounds with.) There have been days where golf was the only thing I talked about and nearly the only thing I thought about, and my non-golfing friends now know way more about the sport than they ever wanted to. I've roped a few into playing with me, too, and actually managed to convert a few to the cause.

I wrote most of this book while living in Durham, North Carolina, a small Southern city where I could drive twenty minutes in almost any direction and hit a golf course. And working on this book was effectively a full-time job, one where cutting out at noon to hit the links technically counted as "research." Now, though, I live in Philadelphia, my home track is a forty-minute drive away, and I have a job that is not writing this book. My golf time is precious, so when I do get to play, each step I take on the course is loaded with intention. I don't even worry about my score, really. Golf is about testing yourself, and my version of that now involves testing the limits of my abilities in any given moment. If I'm faced with a long dogleg right, I'm going to try to hit a drive that curves along with the trees. If it's windy, I might try to keep all my shots low and trending left. If I've got a short approach shot, I figure out which pitch, chip, or flop will be the most difficult and rewarding to pull off and try to make it happen.

Often, this stuff blows up in my face, but after so much golf, it's easy to laugh off. I can always try again, or better yet, try something even more ridiculous now that I'm totally screwed. The trunk of my car is full of random golf clubs, and I love swapping them in and out of my bag just to see how I play with them. This is an objectively terrible way to approach the game if you want to have a good score—and in the appendix of this book, in which I offer some quick tips for going from being a nongolfer to being a golfer, I am going to recommend the opposite of what I do—but it's what I'm personally into at the moment, and I love it. It's the way I've chosen to engage with golf right now, and as long as it's fun for me, I'll stick with it.

There are, truly, so many ways to enjoy golf. There are people whose only interaction with the game is going to the driving range and seeing how far they can smack their driver. There's a dude I follow on Instagram who invented his own form of urban golf involving hitting foam block–looking things at different targets. In Japan, where space is at a premium, nearly three-quarters of a million people play a variation of the game called "park golf," where the holes are extremely short and you need only one club. There are people who play only par 3 courses and are wizards with two wedges and a putter, yet have never so much as touched a fairway wood or a driver. You figure out what works for you and run with it.

Because here is the thing: Your score does not matter. Not in the least. You have no idea how many times I've ruined a perfectly good round because of my perception that I was hitting the ball poorly, and that the person I was playing with was going to think I was somehow unworthy. But nobody cares what you shoot or how you play, because we're all just out on the course trying to do our best. Besides, I've never judged others for how they've played; instead, I'm usually more interested in what they have to say while playing with me.

People have fascinating stories, if you're willing to listen to them. On the first tee of a course in North Carolina, I once met an older guy with a distinct gait who I quickly discovered drove his cart wherever he damn well pleased. We hit our drives, mine down the middle and his not much farther behind, and started making small talk. He asked what I did; I told him I was writing a book about golf and that it was called *How Golf Can Save Your Life*.

"No shit! It saved mine, man!" he said before whacking his shot straight onto the green. He'd grown up in Brooklyn, became an assistant golf pro at one of the top courses in the nation, and even played professionally a bit over in Asia. He'd worked as a plumber for extra cash, and one day he was up on a ladder fixing a pipe in a ceiling when the ladder gave way, sending him straight down to the floor, where he landed directly on his ass. It was a long, hard fall, he said, and when he woke up, he was in a hospital bed with a doctor in his face telling him he was never going to walk again.

I don't know the first thing about science or medicine, but I know honesty and I know when to believe a person's potentially unbelievable story, so I trust he was telling me the truth when he said that he loved golf with every ounce of his being, that it gave him a purpose, and he was not ready to just let go of it because some doctor said so. “I willed myself back to walking so I could play again,” he told me. “I can’t feel shit below my neck, but I’ve still got golf, baby!” He was being modest. He didn’t just have golf. He was the best golfer I’d ever met.

APPENDIX A: HOW TO PLAY GOLF 101

AT A CERTAIN point, it struck me that some of the nongolfers who went to all the trouble of reading an entire book about golf might be interested in actually learning how to play it. If you are one of these people, please enjoy this quick and dirty guide to getting into the game.

We're not going to worry about the rules right now, because honestly, following them will only make you hate golf. You're going to hit a lot of bad shots and lose a bunch of balls when you first start, and so you shouldn't keep track of your score or try to follow up on your terrible shot just yet. At this point in your golf journey, the rules will also make your round of golf slower than it needs to be, and this could leave you and the other people on the course deeply unhappy.

Part One: What You Need and Where to Buy It

In order to play golf, one must possess some golf clubs, a bag in which to hold the golf clubs, some balls, a glove, and some shoes. Of these, the shoes and glove are the most optional—you can just use any athletic shoes to start out, and people get by fine without a glove.

However, the glove exists to keep your hands from blistering, and the shoes will help you grip the ground, and besides, you're about to learn how you can get all this stuff for cheap right now.

Are you near a thrift store? Great, go there and see how much of this stuff you can buy. Depending on the store, you may be able to buy everything you need there, or you might have to keep searching. If you've exhausted the thrift store's stock, check out a used sporting goods store like Play It Again Sports, which will definitely have what you need. Another option: Most golf shops, both stand-alone ones and pro shops connected to golf courses, have a bargain bin section, where you can get used clubs for cheap. All of this will be an adventure, and you will enjoy it.

Part Two: A More Precise Idea of What You're Looking For

Buy the cheapest golf balls you can. Some thrift stores sell a dozen balls in a ziplock bag for a dollar, and almost everyone sells individual used balls for a dollar a pop. Golf Galaxy sells comically large buckets of crappy balls for $20, too. (And most of them are spherical!) The type of ball does not matter for now, as long as they're relatively round and not cracked. You'll probably need about fifty or so to start, and you also might want to snag some plastic or foam practice balls while you're at it, especially if you'd like to hit golf balls in a park.

Your glove should be worn on your nondominant hand and fit snugly; ideally, it will feel like a reassuring hug. Your shoes should be worn on your feet and fit like shoes. I prefer mine to be as small as I can get away with, but you do you. You will almost definitely be able to buy golf shoes at a thrift store, and you can buy a cheapo glove from any golf shop for ten bucks, tops.

If your local thrift store also sells cheap golf bags, you should buy one. If it doesn't, feel free to improvise—I once knew someone who stored his clubs in one of those thin canvas bags you're supposed to carry folding chairs in. You could also just carry the clubs in your hands, because you will not have a lot of them.

Specifically, you need six: a driver, a fairway wood or hybrid, a middle-ish iron like a six-iron, a shortish iron like a nine-iron, a wedge, and a putter. If you're starting from absolute zero, that's going to be more than enough to get you around the course. And more importantly, each is representative of a different type of shot. The driver is for your tee shots; the fairway wood or hybrid is for hitting balls off the ground for long distances; the six-iron is for slightly less long shots off the ground; the nine-iron is for even shorter ones; the wedge is for making precise shots around the green; the putter is for putting.

When picking out your first golf clubs, the ideal ones will cost as close to zero as possible. However, within this constellation of cheapo clubs, there are still certain things you should know:

Your driver should have at least 10.5 degrees of loft, be made of metal rather than wood, and have a large head. Manufacturers have been giving their drivers the maximum legal volume of 460 cubic centimeters for the past fifteen years or so, and you will absolutely be able to find some big, ugly thing that will make a horrifying sound when it strikes a golf ball. Most drivers will be sort of roundish, but for a while there, companies also made drivers that looked like squares. Try to buy a square-shaped one. Technically, its shape may help you, but mainly, they just look fun.

When picking between a fairway wood and a hybrid, you should go with whichever appeals to you visually. If you decide you'd like a fairway wood, avoid getting a three-wood, as it's difficult to make it do the job you will need it to do, which is to hit the ball a long way off the ground. Instead, opt for a five- or seven-wood, which will have seventeen to twenty-one degrees of loft. If you decide you think that a hybrid looks better, try to find one with twenty-one to twenty-three degrees of loft. They make hybrids whose appearances range from that of a miniature fairway wood to that of a beefed-up iron; you should pick one that looks fairway wood-y. Keep in mind that every degree of a club's loft translates to a little less force you will have to impart upon the ball to get it off the ground, but it will also translate to a little less distance. Regardless of its loft, however, your fairway wood or hybrid will soon be your best friend. It's easy to hit and easy to swing, and watching your golf ball fly far into the distance will make you feel satisfied even when it goes in the wrong direction.

When selecting your two irons, you don't have to find ones that are the same model of club from the same company. You'll use the six-iron for a combination of precision and distance, while the nine-iron should be mainly for precision. Try to find ones that aren't just a big block of metal but instead make a big show of distributing the club's weight throughout the head. This might take the form of a cavity scooped out of the back of the iron, or chunky, perimeter-weighted edges. Compare a few different irons with the number "six" and "nine" stamped on them, and you'll start to notice the differences. These, too, will have clubheads that come in different sizes, and as I previously recommended for your driver, try to find one that's on the bigger side of the spectrum.

As for the wedge, you want one with a *lot* of loft, which will allow you to pop the ball up high and have it land soft. Fortunately, most wedges have their lofts stamped on their heads somewhere. Yours should be a sand wedge, which will be about fifty-four to fifty-six degrees—go below that and the ball won't go high enough, but if your wedge has more loft than that, then it's likely that you'll accidentally slide the wedge completely under the ball when you're swinging at it, which will make you feel silly. You may also find a sand wedge that just has the letter "S" stamped on it, in which case, great, problem solved.

When selecting a putter, go nuts. They can be either thin or fat, and their shafts can be either short or long. Used sporting goods stores tend to have a ton of weird, fun-looking putters from throughout golf's history for sale, usually for $10 or less. There are no hard-and-fast rules for selecting a putter, other than that it should make you smile.

One last note: Each golf club has a shaft whose properties give it a unique feel. This is referred to as a shaft's "flex," and in time, it will become very important to have the correct one. Additionally, the golf industry's flex standards are based on antiquated notions of gender and age: The softest shafts are frequently referred to as "Ladies Flex," and the second-softest shafts tend to be called "Senior Flex," although some companies are getting away from this and coding these softer shafts with numbers or letters. The point is, as a beginner, you should avoid clubs whose shafts have things like "Stiff," "X," or "Tour Flex" printed on them, because these are superfirm shafts that will be very difficult for you to hit. Anything else will be fine, honestly.

Part Three: The Grip

Your dominant hand should be positioned lower on the rubber grip than your other hand, and you shouldn't stack them as if you were holding a baseball bat. I mean, I know people who do that, but it's kind of weird. If you've got big hands, you should overlap your dominant pinky and nondominant index finger so that the index rests on the rubber under the pinky; if you have smaller hands, interlock those fingers instead. Regardless of which pinky business you go with, tuck your nondominant thumb into your dominant palm so that you create a little pocket between your palm and the club's grip. This will promote your cradling the grip with the creases of your fingers, the ones at the first knuckle, which will allow your wrists to move freely as you swing. I realize all of that may be difficult to visualize since I haven't included any illustrations, but you can probably find some pictures on Google.

Part Four: The Stance

When you're hitting a golf shot, you should aim to feel your weight resting on the balls of your feet. Some people say you should feel it in your shoelaces, but it's the same principle. You're going to want your feet about shoulder width apart on most shots, but try to space them a little farther apart when you hit your driver and a little closer together when you hit your wedge. You're going to want to have your knees bent a bit, your butt sticking out some, your torso pointed forward, and your neck as aligned with your spine as you can make it. Later, you may want to slightly angle one or both of your feet out away from your body, but let's not get ahead of ourselves.

If all of this feels unnatural, I'm sorry. This may be because I'm doing a bad job of describing it, but do me a favor and try doing it while holding a golf club with that grip I told you about. Position your hands with the club about a fist's worth of distance away from your zipper, so that your arms hang naturally with a slight bit of bend in the elbow. That feels less unnatural, right? You want to put yourself in a position where you allow your body to twist and untwist while maintaining your balance, with the club serving as the counterbalance. Even though it looks like golfers are swinging like hell with their arms, they're actually just creating torque with their torsos. This is a secret.

Go in front of a mirror and hold your golf club using the grip you've just learned while standing in the stance you have also just learned. Make any necessary adjustments to your grip or stance so that everything feels and looks symmetrical. Feel the energy of all things around you, especially your golf club, and listen for the hidden vibrations that hum when we're not paying attention. Is your golf club saying anything to you? If not, whisper the words, "I want to play golf," in a voice that you think a golf club might use, and pretend that the golf club has just spoken.

Part Five: The Swing

Are you near a driving range? If not, that's OK. You can go into a yard or a park. Anywhere, really, where there's grass and space to swing. All you need at this point is your six-iron, which is paradoxically most representative of the rest of the clubs you own and probably the club you'll end up using the least once you actually start playing.

Take the six-iron and grip it with your dominant hand from the incorrect end—the end of it that's usually supposed to hit the golf ball. Assume your golf stance. Put your other hand across your chest until it's touching your opposite shoulder, so that you'll feel your body move once you start doing the next thing that I want you to do.

Here is the next thing: Bring your right hip back, and let everything else follow its lead. You should feel most of your weight on the ball of your dominant foot and a bit of stretch in your butt on the rear side. Don't intentionally move your dominant arm, but notice how it cocks your hand skyward without your having to ask it to. If your nondominant heel wants to lift off the ground, let it. It doesn't have to, but it's OK if it does. After a beat, let go. Do this, I don't know, five more times, just to get a sense of the motion of your backswing.

Now, do this process a seventh time, but once you hit that point of stretching, take the energy you've built up with your twist into an untwist that ends once you've transferred your weight to your front foot. If you do this correctly, your chest will be pointing ninety degrees away, on a horizontal axis, from where it originally was pointing (in other words, to the left if you're right-handed) and your dominant foot will be off the ground, as if you had begun the process of taking a step forward. You can let the hand holding the golf club do whatever it wants, but to a certain degree, it will probably whip the club around your body with a *whoosh*. Once you're comfortable with this motion, see if you can make your club-holding-hand make the same motion that you might if you were throwing a ball underhanded.

It's time to do this all over again, but with your nondominant hand holding the club from the wrong end. This time, just try to keep the club stable as you go through the twisting-and-untwisting process, and don't bend or unbend your elbow too much. Because: Your dominant hand serves as the club's motor, and the nondominant hand is there to ensure stability. The fact that your body is also being used as a motor to drive this whole process might be confusing, and that is probably golf's fault, and also mine.

OK! Time to turn the club the right way and swing with both hands, but do not try to hit a golf ball yet. Instead, think about the good things that would happen if you were actually hitting a golf ball. This will help build up a sense of optimism that will hopefully stay with you once you actually start hitting golf balls. While doing all of this, attempt to keep your head still. Notice the word "attempt" here; you're never going to keep it completely still, but it's still an ideal to hope for, like fully automated disco space communism or a good new *Star Wars* movie.

Once you are comfortable swinging the club and feel optimistic enough to not be completely let down if you screw up and whiff, try actually hitting a golf ball (or, if you're in a park, your foam or plastic practice balls). Place it on the ground, then take your stance so that the ball itself is in the middle of your feet, perhaps a hair toward your front foot. Make sure you're far enough away from the ball that you can swing freely and comfortably, just like you've practiced. Here is a diagram I made using text:

```
                C
                L
          BALL  U
                B

FRONT                     REAR
FOOT                      FOOT
```

OK, so remember all the stuff you just learned in the span of a few paragraphs? Try to think about none of it, but also, make sure you do all of it. The results will probably be disastrous, but this is why you filled up your bucket of optimism from the well of good vibes prior to attempting to strike a golf ball with your golf club. Whatever ends up happening, shake it off. That was a few seconds ago, but you are living in the now. Take a practice swing and try hitting another ball. Repeat this process until you've had enough, and then repeat the process of repeating the process a few times until you've had enough of that. If none of this works, just kind of slap at the ball and be happy that you tried. Now you are ready to go play golf.

Part Six: But Wait!

I'm sorry, I was lying to you. You are now ready to find a course at which you will eventually play golf, because it will have a putting green, where you will practice putting and chipping.

Part Seven: What to Look For in a Golf Course

If you've never played before, then you really need to look for two things: close and cheap. These are still two of the main things I look for in a golf course. Don't worry if the place is crowded or not, because you're going to be playing really slowly.

Once you have picked your cheap and close golf course, take a butt load of balls, your putter, your wedge, and your nine-iron, and head to the practice green.

Part Eight: How to Putt

Putting is, frustratingly, both the most important part of golf and also the least fun. Or at least that's what I used to think, until I suddenly got kind of OK at it. There's no single putting technique that works for everyone, but generally, most people putt using more or less the same setup that they use to hit a regular golf shot.

However!

You should be standing up a bit straighter than you have been when holding your six-iron. This is because a putting stroke is not a body twist but instead a gentle rocking of the upper arms, equal part back, equal part forth, arms relaxed but stable, with your elbows bent to whatever degree feels natural for you. Think about stability through the stroke. Think about the symmetry between all things. Think about how you're about to be good as hell at putting.

You will find that putts roll at different speeds on different greens. In time, you may find that you prefer faster greens to slower ones or vice versa. We're getting ahead of ourselves, though. If this is your first time on a golf course—which, for the purposes of this appendix, I am assuming is the case—then this practice green is the only green that exists. The rest may be out there, but for now, they are Schrödinger's greens.

There are two types of putts you should know about: ones that are three feet from the hole or closer, and ones that are not. The goal is to turn the latter into the former and then sink the former. Take a bunch of your golf balls and set them up in a circle, each in a three-foot radius from a hole, spaced far enough apart that you aren't in danger of stepping on any of them.

Pick a ball, squat behind it, and squint. This is really important. See if there are any subtle curves in the ground that might affect the path of your ball as it makes its way toward the hole. If you're having trouble imagining it, think about what would happen if you spilled a cup of water on the ground and it trickled toward the hole. That's how your ball will travel if you putt it purely. If you're still having trouble visualizing anything at all, you should keep with this pre-putt routine because squatting is supposed to be really good for your back.

Once you have a sense of how the ball will roll, you should imagine the amount of force you'll need to putt it with for it to go in the cup. Keep in mind that the ideal missed putt is one that ends up eighteen inches past its target, so you want to err slightly on the side of more force than less. But if you're new to this stuff, just putt it and see what happens. That's to establish a baseline. If the ball goes in, great. If it doesn't, even better, because now you've given yourself some more information that you can use to make the next one go in.

Putt all the balls in the circle, then keep making golf ball circles around the cup until you get bored or putt an entire circle's balls into the cup. Whichever comes first, really.

As for learning longer putts, there are two ways to do it. One, you can do the circle thing again but increase the radius to four feet, then five, then seven, then ten. Even an inch will add a degree of difficulty to your task, so don't be discouraged if these bigger circles are more difficult. Eventually, the circle will get so wide that the circle game is no longer fun.

Now you can play a new game: Take a golf ball, place it at some random point on the practice green, and visualize your three-foot circle around the hole you'd like to putt it into. Do the squatting thing, imagine water flowing toward the hole (if it's an uphill putt, imagine water flowing down from the hole toward you), and try to make it into the circle. If you successfully do this and then make the following putt, you win. If you miss the big circle, go to wherever the ball is and try putting it into the big circle again. Then try to putt the ball into the hole. No matter how many tries this takes, you are still a winner to me as long as you don't give up.

Part Nine: The Short Game

For a short guide to the short game, please refer to Chapter Seven, which contains my old golf teacher Jimmy's advice on how to hit the bump-and-run. This is the only short game shot you should attempt at this point. Generally, you'll want to use your sand wedge to hit short bump-and-runs and the nine-iron to hit long ones. In the event that your ball needs to fly over an obstacle like a hill or a bush, just pick it up and gently toss it wherever you'd like it to land. If anyone you're playing with says something, remind the person that you just started playing golf, you're not even keeping score yet, and you're just here to have fun. It's possible, though unlikely, that the player will respond in a combative manner; in situations such as these, try lying motionless on the ground until the person goes away, as it is theorized that the eyes of a physically aggressive golfer can detect only objects in motion.

As an added bonus, if you ever lose confidence in your ability to hit solid shots while playing a round, just take your fairway wood or hybrid and hit an overexaggerated version of a bump-and-run. It'll make the ball travel a hundred yards or so on a very low and very straight path, and unlike most things in golf, it's almost impossible to mess up.

Part Ten: Sand Shots

Honestly, I hate sand shots. If your ball lands in a sand trap, just take it out and hit it off the grass. At some point, you'll definitely want to learn how to hit a proper sand shot, just as you'll want to hit a short shot that goes high, but if you end up really enjoying golf, then you should get some lessons.

OK, that's it! Now you are ready to go pro at golf.

APPENDIX B: TERMINOLOGY

Scoring

Par: The score that you're intended to get on any given hole. Generally speaking, there are par 3s, par 4s, and par 5s. It should take you one shot plus two putts to get par on a par 3; two shots plus two putts for a par 4, and three shots plus two putts for a par 5. (By the way, both shots and putts are called "strokes.") Golf courses also have a course par, which is each hole's individual par added up. An eighteen-hole course is divided into a front nine and back nine, each of which usually has a par of 36 which adds up to a total par of 72, but sometimes a course's overall par is a little higher or lower.

Birdie: Whatever par on a hole is, if you score one less than it, then you've just made a birdie.

Bogey: Whatever par on a hole is, if you score one more than it, then you've just made a bogey. If you shoot two shots over par on a hole, then it's a double bogey. Three shots over is a triple bogey, and so on and so forth.

Eagle: Weirdly, there's no such thing as a "double birdie." Instead, two shots under a hole's par is an eagle. To give you a sense of how rare eagles are: I am extremely average at golf and get at least a birdie every month or two; meanwhile, I have gotten an eagle only once in my life and it was due to blind luck.

The Parts of a Golf Hole

Tee Box: This is where you start the hole. It's where you get to tee the ball up to give yourself the best chance of having a good shot.
Fairway: What comes after the tee box. The grass is short and easy to hit off of. Being in the fairway is good. It's what you're aiming for from the tee box if you're playing a par 4 or 5.
Green: What comes after the fairway. It's got the shortest grass, and also the actual hole in the ground where your ball has to go into. You putt on it.
Rough: This is the tall grass that's to the left and right of the fairway. While a fairway is always short, the length and thickness of the rough is left to the golf course's discretion. Some courses make their rough really fun and forgiving, while others let their rough grow so thick that hitting a shot out of it becomes really challenging.
Fringe: What the rough is to the fairway, the fringe is to the green. It's usually less crazy to hit out of than the rough, but after two or three feet of fringe surrounding the green, the fringe gets longer and is the rough again.
Bunkers, aka Sand Traps: These are, as you may have guessed, big pits full of sand. You have to use a special technique to hit out of them, and even a good shot out of the sand is somewhat

unpredictable. Courses usually place bunkers around the green to both increase the difficulty of a hole and to make you, personally, sad. However, they sometimes also place bunkers adjacent to the fairway, or even in it, also to make you sad. The golf course places rakes in sand traps, and after you've hit your sand shot, you're supposed to use those rakes to smooth everything over before you move on. Bunkers are also referred to as "hazards," but there is another type of hazard that I'll tell you about now.

Water Hazards: There is a joke, probably, that the main hazard of golf is playing at all. However, water hazards are ponds, lakes, or creeks placed on a golf course. Unlike a sand trap, you can't really hit out of the water—even the pros rarely try. Instead, you have to take a penalty stroke, drop a ball, and move on with your life. Interestingly, certain courses are beginning to designate places where a pond or whatever *could* be as hazards, in order to cut down on water usage, so in the future, "water hazards" could just be certain parts of the golf course that somebody painted blue. Until then, it'll always be worth taking a minute or two to check the edges of a water hazard to see if you can fish out other people's lost golf balls.

Penalty Areas: Often, the extreme edges of a hole are marked with either red or white stakes. If the stakes are red, that means if your ball goes past them, then you can drop a new ball, take a single penalty stroke, and hit as if the whole imbroglio never happened. If you hit your ball past the white stakes, however, you're in trouble. White stakes signify Out of Bounds; they mean you have to take a penalty stroke *and* hit your ball from its original location—effectively a two-stroke penalty.

The Different Clubs

Driver: This is the big bubble-shaped club that you hit almost exclusively from the tee box. It makes the ball go really far and is fun to hit. Most people carry only one driver.

Fairway Woods: They're shaped like drivers but are way smaller. They can hit a ball off a tee on the tee box, or they can be used to hit a ball off the ground. They can hit a ball pretty far, but not as far as a driver. People usually carry one or two fairway woods.

Hybrids: Also known as utility clubs. These look like a combination of a fairway wood and an iron (see below). They make the ball go fairly far, and are supposed to be easy to use. People usually carry one or two hybrids.

Irons: These make up the bulk of a set of golf clubs and are generally what pops into a person's mind when they think *golf club*. They kind of look like shovels, but with the head of the shovel bent at an angle of almost ninety degrees. Most people carry a five-iron, a six-iron, a seven-iron, an eight-iron, a nine-iron, and a pitching wedge, all of which come in a matching set. The lower the number of an iron, the farther you can hit a ball with it; the higher the number (or if it's a pitching wedge), the shorter you'll hit a ball with it. People used to carry four-irons, three-irons, and, occasionally, two- and one-irons, but it's hard to hit a good shot with a club like that, so most golfers stopped using them once someone invented hybrids.

Wedges: These are like irons, but they're used for hitting the ball *really* short distances. A pitching wedge usually—but not always—matches the rest of a person's iron set and is basically just an iron. After that comes the gap wedge, which is meant for *really really* short shots; then the sand wedge, which, in addition to being optimal for hitting out of a sand trap, allows for *really really really* short shots; and the lob wedge, which, in addition to hitting *really really really really* short shots, also can be occasionally used to hit out of the sand. You also use wedges to hit various shots around the green, including bump-and-runs, chips, pitches, and flops. Bump-and-runs are really low, while chips and pitches are of medium height, and flops are really high.

Putter: This is what you use for mini-golf, and also when your ball is on the green while playing regular-size golf.

Other Golf Terms That Might Be good to Know, Presented in (Mostly) Alphabetical Order

Approach Shot: Any shot that you're hitting in the hope of landing your ball on the green.

Backswing: The first part of the golf swing where you're taking the club back.

Chunk: A misstruck shot where your club hits the ground before it hits the ball. It makes a *chunk* sound, sort of. Actually, it doesn't, but whatever.

Skulled Shot: A mishit involving the bottom of your golf club hitting the ball at its midpoint or even higher, causing your shot to go lower than you had intended, and usually further.

Clubhead: The overall part of the golf club that hits the golf ball.

Clubface: The side of the clubhead that hits the ball.

Shaft: The stick that your clubhead is attached to.

Dogleg: A hole that, rather than leading straight from the tee box to the green, curves either to the left or right.

Draw: A shot that, as it flies through the air, drifts slightly in the direction of the golfer's butt. (Goes from right to left for a right-handed golfer, and from left to right for a lefty.)

Fade: A shot that, as it flies through the air, drifts slightly away from the direction of the golfer's butt. (Goes from left to right for a right-handed golfer, and from right to left for a lefty.)

Hook: Like a draw but bad. For a right-handed golfer, a hook drifts off to the left and then keeps going in that direction until it lands and the golfer has begun to seriously consider quitting the game forever.

Slice: Like a fade but bad. Has all the effects of a hook but instead of going to the left for a right-handed golfer, it goes to the right. Generally speaking, a slice is considered more difficult to fix than a fade.

Greens Fee: The cost to play at a golf course.

Handicap: A number representing how good at golf you are. It's more complicated than that, but that's the gist.

Holing Out: Finishing the hole by getting your ball in the cup. Usually, people only mention "holing out" if they chip their ball in the hole or something similar, rather than simply holing out by putting.

Links: This refers to a specific type of golf course modeled after the ones in Scotland, but it can also be used to refer to a generic golf course.

Lie: The position of your golf ball on the ground relative to where your feet are.

Loft: The angle that your clubface makes relative to its shaft. The driver has the least loft, usually about 8 to 12 degrees, while the lob wedge has the greatest loft, ranging from 58 to 64 degrees.

The lower the loft of a club, the farther it makes the ball go. The higher the loft, the higher it will make the ball go at the expense of distance.

Mulligan: If you hit a really bad shot, sometimes you will declare that it doesn't count and take a do-over. This do-over is called a mulligan. It's technically against the rules, but anyone you're not playing for money with would be a pedant for saying you couldn't take one.

Punch Shot: When, like me, you often find your ball in the woods or some other inconvenient location, you need to hit a low shot that goes a fairly long way. This is called a punch shot, and while it doesn't make up for hitting a good shot in the first place, it can make bad shots hurt less.

Scratch Golfer: Shorthand for someone who's fantastic at golf. Technically this refers to someone with a handicap of zero, but people (including me) throw it around more liberally than that.

Starter: This is a person employed by a golf course to regulate the flow of golfers about to begin their rounds. They are the traffic cop of the golf world, and their word is law.

WORKS CITED

INTRODUCTION

"Golf Preventative Against the 'Flu'." *Evening Capital News* (Boise, Idaho), February 9, 1919. Quoted in "Idaho History: Idaho 1918–1920 Influenza Pandemic," part 32, "Idaho Newspaper Clippings, February 7–13, 1919," *Yellow Pine Times*, November 22, 2020. yellowpinetimes.wordpress.com/2020/11/22/idaho-history-nov-22-2020/.

Kohlstedt, Kurt. "Peewee Urbanism: Why Miniature Golf Grew Big During the Great Depression." 99% Invisible. October 11, 2020. 99percentinvisible.org/article/peewee-urbanism-how-miniature-golf-got-big-during-the-great-depression/.

McCabe, Jim. "How Golf Has Handled Previous Global Crises." PGATour.com. March 31, 2020. www.pgatour.com/news/2020/03/31/how-golf-has-handled-previous-global-crises-spanish-flu-coronavirus-world-war.html.

Stachura, Mike. "The Numbers Are Official: Golf's Surge in Popularity in 2020 Was Even Better Than Predicted." *Golf Digest*, April 7, 2021. www.golfdigest.com/story/national-golf-foundation-reports-numbers-for-2020-were-record-se.

Thomas, Ian. "Golf's Growth in Popularity Is Much Bigger Than a Pandemic Story." CNBC Evolve. September 26, 2021. www.cnbc.com/2021/09/26/callaway-dicks-sporting-goods-score-with-growth-of-golf.html.

CHAPTER TWO

"A Brief History of Revisions to the Rules of Golf: 1744 to Present." USGA.org. March 1, 2017. www.usga.org/rules-hub/rules-modernization/text/a-brief-history-1744-to-present.html.

"Alumni Profile: Wu Linqi." *New York Institute of Technology Magazine*. Accessed August 19, 2022. www.nyit.edu/box/profiles/alumni_profile_wu_linqi.

Gallez, Freddy, and Nijs, Geert. *CHOULE: The Non-Royal but Most Ancient Game of Crosse*. Revised and expanded edition. Published privately, 2021. "The Crosse" chapter accessed at https://ancientgolf.dse.nl/pdfs/crosses%20E.pdf.

McClelland, John. "The History of Golf: Reading Pictures, Viewing Texts." Review of *Golf Through the Ages: Six Hundred Years of Golfing Art*, by Michael Flannery and Richard Leech. *Journal of Sport History* vol. 33, no. 3 (2006): 345–357.

Nijs, Sara. "Fact-finding on 'Jeu de Mail' (Pall Mall): Marseille." *golfika* 25 (Spring 2020): 23–25.

"Rules of Golf as It Is Played by the Society of St. Andrews Golfers." Ruleshistory.org. www.ruleshistory.com/rules1812.html#9.

Vamplew, Wray. "Concepts of Capital: An Approach Shot to the History of the British Golf Club before 1914." *Journal of Sport History* 39, no. 2 (2012): 299–331.

Williamson, John. "The Origins of Golf in Scotland." Chapter 1 in *Born on the Links*. New York: Rowman & Littlefield, 2018.

Yan, Gui, et al. "The Study of Chui Wan, a Golf-like Game in the Song, Yuan, and Ming Dynasties of Ancient China." *Journal of Sport History* vol. 39, no. 2 (2012): 283–297.

CHAPTER THREE

"The Rules of Golf for 2019." R&A Rules Limited and United States Golf Association. www.usga.org/content/dam/usga/images/rules/rules-modernization/golf-new-rules/Rules%20of%20Golf%20for%202019%20(Final).pdf.

Waters, Frank. *The Book of the Hopi*. New York: Penguin Press, 1977.

CHAPTER FOUR

Acker, Kathy. "Against Ordinary Language: The Language of the Body." Published 1993. www.yvonnebuchheim.com/uploads/1/7/0/8/17088324/acker-kathy_the_language_of_the_body.pdf.

Baudelaire, Charles. "The Painter of Modern Life." Written in 1860. In *The Painter of Modern Life and Other Essays*. Translated and edited by Jonathan Mayne. New York: Phaidon Press, 1964.

Foucault, Michel. "Technologies of the Self." Lectures at the University of Vermont, October 25, 1982. foucault.info/documents/foucault.technologiesOfSelf.en/.

"Magazine Audience Measurement: Its Evolution and Pitfalls." *Magazine Dimensions,* 2006. www.mediadynamicsinc.com/uploads/2015/05/magazine_audience_measurements—IY.pdf.

Odell, Jenny. *How to Do Nothing: Resisting the Attention Economy.* New York: Melville House, 2019.

CHAPTER SEVEN

Winogrond, Joseph. "On the Anarchist Origins of Golf." *Fifth Estate* #392 (Fall/Winter 2014). www.fifthestate.org/archive/392-fallwinter-2014/anarchist-golf/.

CHAPTER EIGHT

2019 Pinehurst Membership Information. www.grandepinesnc.com/uploads/1/1/0/7/110764519/2019_pinehurst_membership_information.pdf.

"A Year of Athletics: A Review of the Past Season's Championships." *Pinehurst Outlook*, December 4, 1915: 2.

Brawley, Edward Allan. "The good doctor, the social engineer, and the golfing gems of California." *California History* 86, no. 1 (2008).

Case, Bill. "Second Act: How socialist politician Robert Hunter made the jump to celebrated golf course architect." *PineStraw Magazine*, January 2020: 83.

Debs, Eugene V. *Letters of Eugene V. Debs, Vol. 1*. Champaign: University of Illinois Press, 1990: 95 and 339.

Dugan, Dennis. *Happy Gilmore*. Universal Pictures, 1996.

Gompers, Samuel. "Robert Hunter's New Dilemma." *American Federationist* (Feb. 1915): 355.

Griffith, William. "Robert Hunter and the Problem of Pauperism." *New York Times*, February 19, 1905.

Hunter, Robert. *The Links*. Originally written in 1926. Dublin, OH: Coventry House Publishing, 2018.

———. "The Power of Unionism." *American Federationist* (Feb. 1915): 104.

———. Untitled memoir. Unpublished. Copy obtained from Indiana Historical Society.

Moss, Richard J. "Constructing Eden: The Early Days of Pinehurst, North Carolina." *New England Quarterly* vol. 72, no. 3 (Sep., 1999): pp. 388–414.

"Purchase Mystic Cottage." *Pinehurst Outlook*, April 5, 1913: 2.

Ramis, Harold. *Caddyshack*. Warner Bros., 1980.

Revell, Jay. "The Promise of Pebble Beach." *G and E Magazine*, August 17, 2018. gandemagazine.com/the-promise-of-pebble-beach/.

"Robert Hunter for Senate." *Pinehurst Outlook*, February 28, 1914: 5. *Outlook* story sourced from Associated Press Dispatch.

"The False Teachers and Their Dupes." *New York Times*, March 30, 1908.

"Travis Loses Golf Final." *New York Times*, April 12, 1914.

Watson, Thomas. "I CHALLENGE." *Watson's Magazine* vol. 3 (1909).

CHAPTER NINE

Ceron-Anaya, Hugo. "An Approach to the History of Golf: Business, Symbolic Capital, and Technologies of the Self." *Journal of Sport and Social Issues* vol. 34, no. 3: 339–358.

Conant, Blake Jeffery. "Bankrupt Golf Courses: An Historical Analysis and Strategies for Rebuilding." MA thesis, University of Georgia, 2013. https://getd.libs.uga.edu/pdfs/conant_blake_j_201305_mla.pdf.

Hueber, David. "The Changing Face of the Game and Golf's Built Environment." PhD thesis, Clemson University, 2012. tigerprints .clemson.edu/cgi/viewcontent.cgi?article=1972&context=all _dissertations.

Limehouse, Frank F., Robert E. McCormick, and Melissa M. Yeoh. "The Private Provision of Public Goods: An Analysis of Homes on Golf Courses." *Journal of Private Enterprise* vol. 27, no. 2 (2012): 103–120.

Strahilevitz, Lior. "Exclusionary Amenities in Residential Communities." Coase-Sandor Working Paper Series in Law and Economics No. 250, University of Chicago Law School, Chicago, IL, 2005. chicagounbound.uchicago.edu/cgi/viewcontent .cgi?article=1199&context=law_and_economics.

CHAPTER TEN

Ciardi, John. "Martin Van Buren Was OK." NPR. March 9, 2006. www.npr.org/templates/story/story.php?storyId=5170008.

Correal, Annie. "Raccoons Invade Brooklyn." *New York Times*, January 3, 2016. www.nytimes.com/2016/01/03/nyregion/raccoons-invade-brooklyn.html.

Lucente, Adam. "Animal kingdom: Raccoons rampant in Marine Park, residents report." *Brooklyn Paper*, May 14, 2018. www.brooklynpaper.com/animal-kingdom-raccoons-rampant-in-marine-park-residents-report/.

Morrissett, Ryan, and Golf.com's course raters. "Top 100 Value Courses in the U.S.: The best courses you can play for $150 or less." Golf.com. August 9, 2021. golf.com/travel/top-100-value-courses-you-can-play-150-less/.

Spivak, Caroline. "Scavengers Unearth Buried History—and Maybe Radiation—at Dead Horse Bay." Curbed. August 25, 2020. www.curbed.com/2020/08/ead-horse-bay-beach-brooklyn-radiation-scavengers.html.

Tolchin, Martin. "Marine Park's Littered Landscape." *New York Times*, April 6, 1965.

Young, Michelle. "The Top 10 Secrets of Marine Park, Brooklyn." Untapped New York. untappedcities.com/2017/03/21/the-top-10-secrets-of-marine-park-brooklyn.

CHAPTER ELEVEN

Dostoyevsky, Fyodor. *Notes from the Underground*. Seattle: AmazonClassics, 2017.

Woods, Tiger, with Daniel Rapaport. "The new tee shot Tiger Woods relies on under pressure, and how you can play it." *Golf Digest*, February 4, 2020. www.golfdigest.com/story/the-new-tee-shot-tiger-woods-relies-on-under-pressure-and-how-y

ACKNOWLEDGMENTS

Writing a book, like playing golf, is simultaneously easy and unfathomably difficult. On one hand, you just start typing and don't stop until you've written a book. On the other hand, there reaches a point very early on in the typing process when fear and/or self-doubt and/or panic starts to seep in, and that tends to make the actual typing very difficult. It would be impossible for me to thank every single person who helped create a protective barrier of confidence and love under which I could type this little book, but just know that if you're reading this and thinking, *Hey wait, why didn't Drew mention me?* then I couldn't have done it without you.

Thanks to my agent, Tina Pohlman, who guided me through this entire process with wit, verve, and, most of all, patience. And to my editor, Samantha Weiner, at Abrams, as well as her colleagues Juliet Dore and Annalea Manalili who taught me to think of this book as a big block of text to improve and polish and spit-shine, and were willing to show me how to make this into the book it wanted to be—and at times, jump in there and mold this book alongside me.

And thanks to my parents, who have encouraged, supported, and believed in me as I've fumbled my way through adulthood. I love you and I'm sorry for all the swears. I promise I took out all the ones that I could.

More thanks: to Kevin Munger, for your notes and sympathetic responses to my stress-texts; Charlie Hulme for always being down to talk through ideas and offering feedback on early chapters amid the walks; Luke Davis and the whole Lie + Loft crew for welcoming me into the Triangle golf scene; everybody at Hillandale in Durham for making their golf course feel like home to anyone who steps on its turf; Troy and Whitaker for gamely consenting to me writing about our golf team; Naomi Zucker for an extremely crucial last minute assist; JJ Lang and James Yeh for allowing me to teach them how to swing a seven-iron and putt a golf ball (respectively); Kim Kelly and Dan Ozzi for showing me that it could be done; Jeremy Gordon, Yannick LeJacq, Kyle Kramer, and Nolan Allan for their endless support and friendship; Orin Starn for guidance in all things on and off the course; the VICE group chat for all the Zoom poker sessions; Brandy Jensen and Willy Staley for editing essays that ended up being key building blocks for this book; and everyone who I've ever met at a party who felt bound by social pressure to politely listen to me talk about golf.

More than anything, I need to thank Emilie Friedlander, whose love, support, and conscientious edits helped this book exist. It is a sign of her never-ending wisdom and heart that she just now reminded me that I needed to thank our dogs, Nora and Percy, and our cat, Leopold, whose antics and purity of soul bring so much joy to our lives.

I'd also like to thank French Montana and Bryan Ferry, because I listened to their music a *bunch* while writing this book, as well as Virginie Despentes, whose Vernon Subutex trilogy gave me a shot of literary adrenaline when writing had me feeling most drained. I've never met any of them, but I'd play golf with them at the drop of a hat.

And finally, thanks to every person I've ever played golf with, each of whom inspired this book in some small way.

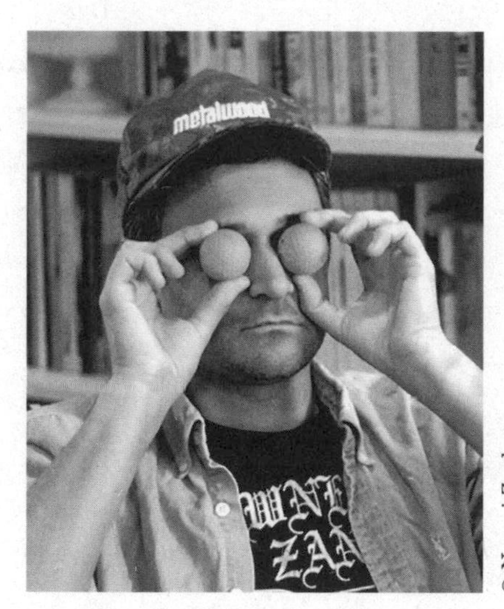
metalwood